SP

Somerleyton Press

Surviving Lyme Disease Using Alternative Medicine

Dr. David A. Jernigan, D.C., B.S.

SP

Somerleyton Press
Wichita, Kansas, USA

SP

Somerleyton Press
545 N. Woodlawn
Wichita,KS, USA

Cover Design by Advanced Technical Graphics, Wichita, Kansas
Printed by Complete Printing, Decatur, Indiana

Manufactured in the United States of America

First Printing: 1999

ISBN 0-967623-0-4

Dedication

This book is dedicated to my lifelong colleague and wife,
Dr. Sara J. Jernigan, B.S., D.C.
Whose scintillating intellect, support, and understanding are outshone only by her love for God and her family;
A woman truly without guile.

Special thanks also to:

Dr. Lida Mattman, Ph.D., whose perseverance and dedication to research is an inspiration and without whom none of this would have come to pass.
Dr. Milton Dowty, my mentor, who set my foundation on a higher mountain; and who gave to me the tools essential to attain higher truths in doctoring.
Dr. Durwin Smith who always patiently listened and brainstormed with me.

Very special thanks to my entire family of patients who pushed me to find new answers, who trusted, and stuck with me through it all.

Disclaimer

All of the facts in this book have been very carefully researched, and many have been drawn from the scientific literature. For obvious reasons, the following does <u>not</u> claim to substitute for a physician's care, nor does it advocate specific solutions to individual problems. The physicians and experts providing the following information have substantiated their claims as well as possible, considering that data on health and nutrition are subject to change as we learn more. These products and the information below should not be regarded as a substitute for professional medical treatment.

Table of Contents

Introduction

This book is intended to present an alternative protocol for CHRONIC Lyme Disease. It is intended for lay people and physicians who desire to supplement their diet and create a more rounded healing regime. One can easily pick up literature about a myriad of vitamins, minerals, botanical medicines, glandulars, homeopathic remedies, enzymes, and colloidal metals and minerals...all promising to "cure" what ails you. I see patients everyday who have been everywhere and tried everything (and many have the bags of remedies to prove it!) The point is, if your bottom-line problem is a bacterial infection and the remedy you are taking is the world's greatest antioxidant...it doesn't matter how much of the antioxidant you take...it is not going to touch the bacterial infection! You must address all of the bottom-line problems.

The protocol presented in this book revolves around two phenomenal products called Borrelogen and Virogen. These two are what I consider to be the central synergistic remedies because they alone address the most bottom-line issues for the majority of people suffering from chronic Lyme Disease. However, no one or two remedies can address all of the problems associated with a multi-system illness. Each of the remedies, supplements and therapies recommended in this book complement each other and have a strong synergistic effect on the entire body.

Antibiotics are a viable tool of your physician. Nothing presented here preempts or implies superiority in killing spirochetes. However, most people with chronic Lyme Disease have already used many antibiotics with limited relief, or may be allergic to them. If you have just been bitten and infected by a tick…definitely seek out a physician who will treat you using appropriate antibiotics. But, if you have chronic Lyme Disease, hopefully you will find a physician who will treat you following a similar path to what I am presenting in this book.

I decided to write this book after seeing so many people suffering using primarily antibiotics. In my office, I rarely recommend that someone use "just" Borrelogen and Virogen. I use many different treatments and therapies, best suited to the patient based on my testing. In my clinic I have over five thousand different remedies from all over the world at my disposal. Based on my experience, I developed what I consider to be the optimum selection of remedies. This protocol gets right down to the business of healing a body as rapidly as possible. I feel that this protocol is the best, most well rounded plan around. It is designed so that anyone suffering from this illness can have the best chance of getting over it.

The concepts and protocol presented in this book is the result of my ongoing research to find and/or develop better remedies and therapies, to help real people, and real suffering in my clinic. I can only treat so many patients in one day at my clinic, but many more people can benefit from my research through this vehicle.

It is difficult to say what would have happened had you or had you not followed this protocol. I feel confident that this protocol will strengthen your body at the very least and give you the best fighting chance of conquering and reclaiming the quality of life you seek.

Keep in mind, not to be morbid, that we are all dying and coming closer to death with the passing of every second. The choices you make either add days to your life or take them away. Suppressive therapies used by themselves, always take days away, since they weaken the tissues of the body. It is your body…it is also your choice.

I pray that you prosper and find good health all the days of your life.

Dr. David A. Jernigan

Chapter 1

The Great Imitator

The "Great Imitator", Lyme disease (LD), is increasingly being confirmed in cases of misdiagnosed chronic illnesses. It is said to be the "great imitator" due to the fact that it can mimic over 200 illnesses. This fact, and the fact that there have been no good laboratory tests available to positively confirm LD, has led to the polarization of the medical and scientific community.

Until recently, the lab tests could only detect the "shadow" or the "possibility" that your body has seen the lyme bacteria, *Borrelia Burgdorferi*, via serum antibody tests. Serum antibody testing, such as the Lyme Western Blot IgG/IgM, in reality does not confirm the actual presence of the Lyme bacteria. The presence of Lyme specific antibody seen in a Lyme Western Blot can arguably be said that your body has simply "seen" this type of bacteria before.

If you had Strep throat, your doctor could perform a throat culture and definitively confirm the presence of the actual Strep bacteria. Also the doctor could test and find that the white blood cell count and neutrophils were elevated, further confirming the strep bacterial infection. The Borrelia burgdorferi is a type of bacteria which can elude your body's immune system; therefore, the lab tests show no elevated white blood cells, or neutrophils. The fact is your body's immune system apparently can not see these bacteria, leading some of the world's Lyme researchers to label the bacteria as a "*Stealth Pathogen*".

One can see why so many otherwise very intelligent doctors have a difficult time acknowledging Lyme disease as a possible diagnosis for their patients. The training that most doctors receive dictates that one must confirm facts with laboratory tests. If it does not show up on lab testing, or if the patient does not fit the profile, then most doctors absolutely will not consider lyme as a possible answer. Thankfully, recent research has determined a culturing method that allows a laboratory to "culture" or grow the spirochete bacteria responsible for Lyme disease. This testing is still in its infancy, but has appeared in scientific peer-reviewed journals. It is hoped that it will soon receive the FDA seal of approval so that it will be included under standard insurance coverage, and more reference laboratories will begin to offer this test.

Lyme Disease, The Great Imitator, may express itself by the following symptoms (although this listing is certainly not all inclusive):

- Rash at bite site or other sites
- Muscle twitching of the face or other areas
- Unexplained fevers, sweats, chills
- Headache
- Fatigue
- Neck creaks and cracks, neck stiffness
- Unexplained weight change — (loss or gain)
- Tingling, numbness, burning, stabbing sensations
- Unexplained hair loss
- Facial paralysis
- Swollen glands
- Eyes/vision: loss of vision, double, blurry, pain, increased floaters
- Sore Throat
- Ears/hearing: buzzing, ringing, ear pain
- Testicular pain/pelvic pain
- Dizziness, poor balance
- Increased motion sickness
- Unexplained menstrual irregularity
- Light headedness, wooziness, difficulty walking

- Unexplained milk production (lactation)
- Tremors
- Irritable bladder or bladder dysfunction
- Disturbed sleep
- Sexual dysfunction or loss of libido
- Confusion, difficulty in thinking
- Upset stomach or change in bowel function
- Difficulty with concentration or reading
- Chest pain or rib soreness
- Forgetfulness, poor short term memory
- Shortness of breath, cough
- Difficulty with speech
- Heart palpitations, pulse skips, heart block
- Joint pain or swelling
- Mood swings, irritability, depression
- Stiffness of the joints, neck, or back
- Heart murmur or valve prolapse
- Muscle pain or cramps
- Exaggerated or worse hangover from alcohol

Chapter 2

Pleomorphism of Lyme Spirochetes

A complication of successful diagnosis and treatment can be appreciated by the fact that Borrelia burgdorferi (Bb) are *pleomorphic* organisms[1]. A pleomorphic organism takes on a different shape at different life stages. A butterfly is said to be pleomorphic because it changes from a caterpillar to a cocoon to a butterfly. The lyme bacteria is known to be pleomorphic. The different pleomorphic stages of Borrelia burgdorferi are unclear, but research suggests that it can definitely exist as *cell-walled bacterium, or cell-wall deficient bacterium* depending on its life cycle. Again, each stage of the cycle is relatively "stealth".

A cell wall is requisite in order for the spirochete Borrelia burgdorferi to achieve its spiral shape. Some antibiotics act to disrupt the mechanisms in the cell wall of the Bb in order to kill the bacteria. It is suspected that the long-term antibiotic attack on the cell walls can cause the spirochete to revert into a *"cell wall deficient"* form as a survival mechanism. The problem is that the Bb can revert back and forth between the classic spiral shape and the cell wall deficient shapes. To complicate matters more the Bb can exist simultaneously as both forms. Dr. Lida Mattman, Ph.D., a leading researcher in L Form bacteria, has found that it is common to see three Lyme spirochetes for every seven Lyme L Forms in a blood specimen. Also, it is not uncommon to see only L Forms with no spirochetes to be found[1].

The cell wall deficient form is synonymously called *L Forms*, and *spheroplasts*. Many different bacteria and fungi can achieve this form. For unification purposes scientists now refer to the cell wall deficient stage as L Forms[2].

It may sound strange that any organism can exist at all without a cell wall. This term can be a little deceiving in that there is a membrane where the cell wall used to be. Without its cell wall, the Bb cannot hold its characteristic spiral shape. It has been speculated that Lyme infected ticks can also harbor the L Form of the Bb, which may explain why not every infected person develops a bulls-eye rash or tests positive on initial blood tests[3]. It may be safely said that every chronically infected LD patient has both spirochetes and L Forms.

Indications are that the Bb can be forced into remission for weeks to years with long term aggressive use of antibiotics. During this remission there are usually no detectable Bb spirochetes and titers go down to undetectable levels. The Bb could possibly be latent in its L Form during this stage. Apparently when the conditions are right the latent L Form infection reverts back to the spirochete form, the symptoms return, and the titers go up, leaving one to wonder if they were bitten again by an infected tick.

Not only does the spirochete change from a cell-walled bacterium to an L-form bacteria but it is possible for each life stage to exist independently from the other stage[2]. Recent research has shown that laboratory animals injected with dead fragments of the classic spirochetal Borrelia burgdorferi contracted Lyme disease[3]. This is significant because bacteria do not replicate themselves from eggs, but from fission. Therefore, a possible explanation might be that the undetected cell wall *deficient* life-stage actually was responsible for these laboratory-induced infections.

Bacterial pleomorphism is not unique to the Lyme bacteria. Treponema pallidum, the bacteria known to cause Syphilis are also widely known to prefer different shapes depending on where they are found in the body[4].

Recently, scientists unlocked the genetic sequencing of the

B. burgdorferi bacteria and found that 50% of its genetic make-up is identical to that of the Syphilis bacteria[5]. Due to the homeopathic law of *similars*, or "likes cure likes", doctors should consider a single dose, or a few doses, of the homeopathic nosode Syphilinum 200c. Upon reading the homeopathic materia medica, one will see a great many similar symptoms of the chronic lyme patient that may be corrected by this one homeopathic remedy. (Miasms are the tendencies and predisposition to certain physical and psychological problems either acquired or inherited due to illness or suppressive treatments)[6].

The ability to change shape is thought to be the reason why the Lyme bacteria, once well established in the body, is able to survive even after long-term antibiotic therapies. It is possible that the Lyme bacteria flip-flop between both shapes to escape the antibiotics. People who receive antibiotic treatment soon after they were infected recover completely, since the organism has not had time to "dig-in" and cycle into the other pleomorphic shapes. The fact that antibiotics only address the bacterial stage may also explain why many people under antibiotic therapy feel improvement while on the antibiotics only to relapse soon after discontinuing the antibiotics.

Those placing their faith in antibiotics to "cure" them of *chronic* Lyme disease will in most cases be disappointed. Drug therapies such as antibiotics address only the offending bacteria but do nothing to heal the body as a whole.

An analogy might be seen in the following example: If you have termites eating their way through the wood of your house, you can call an exterminator to spray harsh chemicals into the wood effectively killing the termites. You have now removed the cause of the problem, but the extermination did nothing to correct the damage already caused. To make matters worse, you now have a toxic substance soaked into the wood of your house.

Lyme disease is a systemic infection affecting your body on every level. Since every organ and tissue is totally integrated and reliant upon each other, any time one system is affected it will ultimately create a chain-reaction of other organs and glands that become progressively dysfunctional the more time goes by. For example, anyone who has suffered with chronic Lyme disease will tell you that the mind and the body are affected over time.

As you can see, if you have chronic Lyme disease, you absolutely take your healing very seriously. You must not rely on your doctor to "cure" you…he only sees you for a few minutes in his treatment room. It is up to you to walk out your healing minute by minute. If your doctor says to take a remedy four times per day, and you only take it two or three times per day, 'because it wasn't convenient to take it four times', or you 'keep forgetting to take it', you are prolonging your illness, and risk making the Lyme organism become drug-resistant. In this case, you will possibly be stuck with it for life. Lyme disease is a war that you fight 24 hours a day.

If you have the Lyme Disease your fight will be easier to fight now that you know the spirochete tends to be pleomorphic. Therefore, one must use a treatment protocol that recognizes the different cycles of this spirochete.

Chapter 3

Borrelia burgdorferi & Mycoplasmal Infections

When the Bb are in their L Form phase, the morphology, or appearance cannot be distinguished from that of Mycoplasma organisms. In fact there is only one primary difference between the two organisms; mycoplasma by definition cannot generate a cell wall[1]. For those of you who are unfamiliar with the term mycoplasma do not feel bad. It is only recently that the pathogenic nature of these organisms have come into the forefront of the medical mindset. A mycoplasma is larger than a virus and smaller than bacteria. Mycoplasma are more closely akin to bacteria than viruses. They are said to be the smallest self-replicating life form[2]. Like Bb these mycoplasma can infect deep tissues and create almost all of the same symptoms as LD[3]. A plethora of research has connected mycoplasmal infections to many of today's most prevalent illnesses such as Lyme Disease, Chronic Fatigue Syndrome (CFS), Fibromyalgia Syndrome (FMS), and even the Gulf War Syndrome (GWS)[4].

How does this impact you?

Any person suffering with chronic LD knows that it is affecting multiple systems of the body. This fact causes a weakened and susceptible immune system. Sufferers of chronic LD/CFS/FMS/GWS become microbe collectors. Your resistance to foreign invaders such as mycoplasma is greatly reduced. When considering the effects of having multiple pathogenic infections at the same time, it is no wonder that so many people undergo years of treatment without complete resolution of their symptoms. It is already well recognized that people suffering from LD may also have other infections going on at the same time, such as Babesia microti, Ehrlichiosis, and Candidiasis. To make matters worse we are now realizing that mycoplasmal infections can be detected in the blood of 60-70% of all LD/CFS/FMS sufferers. "Systemic mycoplasmal infections are a major source of morbidity in CFS, FMS, and Gulf War Illness patients, and they need to be treated with antibiotics…and nutritional support"[5].

When considering the fact that the Bb can also revert to a mycoplasmal look-a-like, L-Form, one can begin to grasp the true difficulties of determining an effective treatment protocol. But do not get disheartened, all of this is treatable! I am simply attempting to educate you so that you can know what you are up against and understand your enemy.

If you have been treated for Lyme Disease, and have reached the point where all of the lab tests indicate that you no longer have any Borrelia burgdorferi, yet you are still feeling very sick; then your doctor needs to do a mycoplasma PCR test on you. Also have him test for the other common co-infections, Babesia microti, Ehrlichia, and systemic candida. If you have never tested positive to having Lyme Disease then definitely get your doctor to test for mycoplasmal infections.

Chapter 4

Borrelia burgdorferi Toxins...The <u>Cause</u> of Your Symptoms?

Research and clinical studies have determined that there is a toxin released by the Borrelia burgdorferi spirochete[1]. Cholera bacteria and others are known to release a toxin. It is this Bb toxin that is likely most responsible for the symptoms experienced by Lyme sufferers. When a doctor uses an antibiotic and kills some spirochetes, there is a resultant Jarish-Herxhiemer reaction...a worsening of the patient's symptoms in response to the increased release of bacterial die-off toxins. The toxins are dumped into the blood stream and are circulated throughout the body until they can either be eliminated by the body or become lodged in areas of weakened tissues. These lodged toxins are one of the reasons that symptoms can persist even after the actual Bb infection is gone, since the toxins can remain as an irritant in the tissues for years.

Our bodies do not have adequate detoxification mechanisms to detoxify these Bb toxins. In theory, if scientists could develop a Lyme anti-toxin, one could have the infection without the symptoms. One problem with this mindset is that many doctors use the Jarish-Herxhiemer (herx) reaction to determine when the prescribed antibiotic is working, i.e. the worse the herx the better the antibiotic is working. Without the herx these doctors have no way of determining if the medicine is working. They do this because most doctors have **not** been trained in Electro-dermal testing, or similar testing techniques that allow the doctor to know when a medicine is working, or if the patient is actually allergic, or toxic to a medication.

Eliminating the toxin would in theory eliminate this worsening of symptoms. Before this elimination can effectively be used by most doctors two things must occur... 1) a better method of testing for the presence or absence of the infection must be implemented. 2) Utilization of Bio-Resonance testing, Electro-dermal testing or similar testing to individualize the selection of medicines for each patient.

The mineral molybdenum can dramatically aid in the detoxification of the toxins created from the dysfunction of multiple tissues in chronic illness. Molybdenum is very useful for detoxifying the toxin, aldehyde, from the die off of candida type yeast. This is important to Lymies due to the fact that aldehydes are considered neurotoxins, or nerve poisons. Aldehydes are also the toxin responsible for the hangover experienced by drinking excessive amounts of alcohol. I know of many Lymies who complain of this hung over feeling without having drunk any alcohol[2]. (However, it is our experience that it will not detoxify the specific Bb toxin.) Even though every Lyme sufferer should use molybdenum to get rid of the aldehyde toxins, they also need to drink plenty of purified water to keep the everyday metabolic toxins flushed out of the tissues. Taking molybdenum will help slow the degeneration of tissues and related symptoms from the toxic overload.

Chapter 5

Getting Rid of the Lyme Disease is More Than Getting Rid of Bacterial Infection

I cannot stress enough the need for your doctor to be addressing all the systems of the body on every visit. The body is totally integrated, and should perform like an orchestra, with every organ and tissue keeping rhythm with all the rest of the body.

If one organ becomes dysfunctional due to illness or trauma, it ceases to move with correct rhythm in relation to the three dimensional movement of the other organs. When this happens it throws off the natural rhythm of the entire body. Eventually no tissue is able to maintain the proper rhythm. It is inevitable that this chain-reaction will occur progressively over time, if left uncorrected.

While it is true that there is usually one offending issue that starts the whole chain-reaction, if left undiagnosed and untreated for very long, the problem will become complicated by the aftereffects of the original cause. Weakened tissues lose their natural resistance to things such as parasitic infection, toxin overload, disregulated chemistry, and fungal and microbial infection.

Let us take the example of Lyme Disease...a person gets bitten by an infected tick and becomes infected with the bacteria known as Borrelia burgdorferi. The bacteria migrate through the tissues making their way to the muscles, joints, connective tissues, organs, the brain and nervous tissues. The bacteria wreak havoc on your body. To let you know that there is something wrong, your body responds with a multitude of symptoms.

If treated early in the infection all is well, but if the infection is not detected and treated immediately then the body's resistance is weakened and the chain-reaction begins.   Like every organism, the Lyme bacteria live a certain life span and then die. This means that even without treatment you will have a certain number of Borrelia burgdorferi bacteria dying-off every few weeks. These dying bacteria end up causing you trouble since they release toxins upon dying (also known as the cause of a Jarish-Herxhiemer reaction). These toxins lodge in the tissues of the body causing a worsening of the symptoms you feel. Research has shown that there is no direct tissue damage from the spirochetes. The damage to tissues is primarily due to the spirochete toxins which increase the inflammatory and immune responses[1]. Here is where the chain reaction begins to be most pronounced.

To examine how this happens let us start with a hypothetical example. Let us say the toxins are primarily affecting the elasticity of your muscles for argument sake. The muscles perhaps of your right leg become tight and cramp, with wandering pains. You begin to favor that leg, walking with a limp. You are not designed to walk in this manner, so structural integrity is compromised. Your body's structural components are now exceeding their design limitations. The knee and hip joints begin to swell in response to the strain. The pelvis becomes unlevel throwing the entire spine into fits attempting to compensate for a tilted pelvis. The pelvis and intervertebral discs of the spine become inflamed from the changes in weight distribution, which in turn irritate the spinal nerves. The spinal nerves are important in carrying the brain's messages for regulating every organ's function. With the spinal nerve irritation comes radiating pains in different areas of the body, tingling, numbness, and loss of control. The organs begin to reflect the spinal problems and cannot get a clear signal from the brain, therefore the chemistry and hormones become dysregulated.

Every organ is on its own dedicated electrical circuit with at least one set of muscles. When there is a problem anywhere in an organ circuit, it causes the entire circuit to become, for all intents and purposes, short-circuited. The damaged organ circuit will only work at about 40% of its normal electrical and functional capacity. This is one of the body's protective mechanisms. The body will "turn down" the available electricity to a damaged area so that you cannot damage it further by still being able to exert 100% energy into an area that needs to be repaired. The decreased energy in one circuit disrupts the rhythm of the organs which, one by one, respond by going into compensation mode and eventually into complete dysfunction. By now, you hurt all over. You have tender spots in the muscles. Your joints take turn aching and hurting. Your brain won't seem to work right, and you can't seem to sleep even though you are completely worn out all day long. It seems like nothing in your body is working correctly. You go to the doctor, who may not believe that Lyme is a problem in your State, but runs other tests, which are "inconclusive", since there is no "real" disease process, only the compensation of tired organs. And the Lyme Disease goes on.

Finally, you found a doctor who determines you have Lyme Disease. "Not a problem", he may say. "Just take this antibiotic and you should be better in six weeks". At the end of six weeks he proclaims you cured, only you don't feel any better or you feel like you are still not well. Did he address everything? Usually all he has addressed is just the infection. That's great! But what about the structural imbalances that have now been there for months or years? How about the organ circuits which didn't magically come back "online"? Did he address the opportunistic parasites, yeast, and viruses that found a home in your body while your resistance was down? How about the toxins stored in the tissues? What about building up the nutrients and jumpstarting the glands of the body so that the body can begin the work of healing itself?

Folks, can you begin to see how difficult it can be to achieve total wellness after a long fight with something terrible such as Lyme Disease? If your doctor is simply giving you antibiotics with the hope that everything will go back to normal as soon as the bacteria is gone…then you need to find a new doctor or find another doctor to cover all the other areas needing healing.

Getting rid of the bacteria in a disease such as Lyme Disease can many times be just the beginning of the fight. You now must rebuild every tissue of your body. This takes time. A general rule of thumb in chronic illness is to expect three months of doing everything right, for every year you have had the problem. This doesn't mean that you won't feel better sooner. It simply means that *feeling good and being healthy are two different things*. Most people diagnosed with cancer or heart disease say they 'never felt better'…their doctor just found the problem in a routine examination. So, be patient with yourself.

Keep a journal so you can see improvement over long periods of time. Rejoice in small triumphs. Control your thinking…don't allow yourself to become depressed. Don't talk about the different symptoms…talk about the things that are better. See yourself *half-well instead of half-sick.* Cooperate with the different doctors and therapists who are trying to help you. Don't be lazy in your mind, rejoice and actively participate in the healing of your body. You cannot afford to just take the pills and live a dark, dismal life, waiting for the pills to work. Change your routines. Strive to be vital in rebuilding your body. You are not a victim; you are simply living life like everyone else…all have problems to deal with. You cannot afford to allow yourself to "become an illness"; this just leads to a rapid decline. The illness is not who you are. Become one with God and one with yourself, not one with the illness. Get outside in the sunshine and close to nature and simplify life so that your priorities are correct. The decisions you make today will determine your tomorrow. Above all control your thinking…it's the one thing God gave you total control over…its your free-will choice to accept or reject the illusions and lies that come to your mind. You can reclaim your quality of life and the journey is the prize.

Chapter 6

Get the Hurt and the Dirt Out of Your Life

A common misconception is for one to say "I was fine before this bug bit me". It may be so, but feeling good does not guarantee that you are healthy. It is my experience that most people have much unresolved hurt and dirt contributing to their state of health. Everyone at any given moment may have as many as two hundred potentially pathological organisms in their body. Why aren't we all sick? Could it be that what we call the human organism has the ability to control every pathological microbe? A totally healthy human does this very thing without you even thinking about it!

I have often wondered at the wide diversity of symptoms that I see in some patients . Lyme does not affect any two people in the exact same way. I have seen people with only one prevailing symptom though positive for LD. There are common symptoms, but there are always many symptoms that fall outside of the norm. As a doctor I have to wonder why the Borrelia burgdorferi spirochete affected the patient in this unique way. From my clinical experience I have come to the conclusion that not only can *chronic* Lyme Disease bring about new problems to your body, but it is unique in that it also brings the dirt of your life to light.

From birth to present time your body is constantly being challenged. These challenges may arise from emotional traumas such as the death of a loved one, physical, sexual and emotional abuse, physical injuries such as auto accidents, chemical challenges from medicines or pollution, not to mention stress from inherited tendencies. Any unresolved issues will be made manifest physically or psychologically as your body becomes more dysfunctional by the chronic infection of LD.

Most people can recall a time when they injured their body. We'll say you injured the back for this example. You may have not ever gone to get it treated, and eventually the pain went away. The body adapted to the problem. The problem is still there, only now the pain and the problem are "put on the back burner" by your brain. This adaptation mechanism of the body occurs on every level, whether the level is of a physical, chemical, or psychological nature. Unfortunately, many times these insults cannot be effectively adapted to and they manifest in an ever worsening cascade of symptoms to get your attention so you can deal with the true cause.

Chronic illness breaks down the body's ability to keep these problems on the "back burner". These back burner problems are areas of weakened tissues, which may have never manifested as an obvious problem if life had gone on without a major challenge such is Lyme Disease. The fact is that the Bb and any other invading organism or parasite will always go to the weakest areas of the body first. This phenomenon is seen throughout nature. One example of this is seen in the plant kingdom. Plants that come from a strong genetic heritage and have been nurtured in ideal conditions for generations, have an increased natural resistance to bugs and plant illnesses. Weak plants from poor soil and poor genetic heritage are extremely susceptible to infections.

The point of all of this is that you are sum total of all of the challenges and lifestyle decisions you've made. In chronic Lyme Disease, all of this will be brought to the fore front and all of it will need to be finally addressed by you and your healthcare team.

Everyone has heard the saying…you are what you eat…well you really are much more than that. You are, more accurately, the sum total of all that you have experienced. You integrate all of the good in your life, and hopefully resolve all of the bad. Anything bad that goes unresolved will affect the entire human organism.

The Bible deals with much of this topic. It says to control your thinking...by taking every thought "captive". We know now from science that whenever you *allow* yourself to become depressed, that every cell in your body becomes hypofunctional, or depressed. We also know that when the Bible says to not let the sun set on our wrath, that perpetuating that negative emotion over night causes an energetic "computer virus" affecting the body in its entirety, in a way unique to the type of negative emotion. So you can see how important it is to exert your free will choice to control your thinking. Thought is the only thing God gave you complete control over in the five senses world. This line of thought may shock many of you, but it must be dealt with, because of all of the perpetuation I hear from patients of unresolved anger, fear, unforgiveness, and the like. God said it, but also medical science has verified it...these issues affect the entire body. The ability of the immune system to function, and the ability for the body to heal itself is directly reflected by the number of unresolved issues. The problem for you and your healthcare team is that many times you had issues that went unresolved that even you have forgotten. Out of sight is not out of mind. Many of these unresolved issues cannot be dealt with using a pill, but they very definitely must be brought to resolution.

- Your greatest avenue and **"First-Aid"**, for correcting these unresolved issues is your one on one communication with your heavenly Father...God. You must let go and resolve any known issues with Him. Having done so...do not look back...let the issues be permanently non-issues. This requires one to completely clean out the "rooms in your mind" where these issues reside. Forgive and forget it. Get rid of the emotion attached to the issue, so that if the issue is brought up again in the future you don't have to go down the emotional path you used to associate with that event. The fact of the matter is that the past does not define who you are today nor does it determine your tomorrow. If you do not know God as your heavenly Father, then seek Him out. (Romans 10:9,10) Having done so, change your habit patterns of thinking. Stop watching your soap operas, or your fishing shows and put your energy into reading God's Word, and into reading self improvement books. Listen to motivational or educational tapes instead of the news. Do volunteer work for worthy causes. Eventually you will maintain an attitude of a conqueror instead of that of a victim.

If you already have a great relationship with your heavenly Father, wonderful. I'll just share with you a few verses, which I find as a doctor interesting. I am always interested in what God says about sickness. In I Corinthians 11:28-30, God mentions why some are sick as He talks about the partaking of communion unworthily...

I Corinthians 11:28-30

But let a man examine himself, and so let him eat of that bread, and drink of that cup. For he that eateth and drinketh unworthily, eatheth and drinketh damnation (condemnation) *to himself, not discerning the Lord's body. For this cause many are weak and sickly among you, and many sleep* (die).

For this cause many are weak and sickly among you, and many have died." Now as a doctor reading this I really take notice, especially when God our Creator Himself says that this is a cause of much illness! I'm in the business of helping people to heal. The next logical question is 'If this is possibly the cause of my sickness, how do I correct it?' God tells us how in the same chapter. In verse 28 He tells us, "...let a man <u>examine</u> himself, and so let him eat of that bread and drink of that cup." Within these verses are the remedy or the medicine for correcting this problem! Drinking and eating communion <u>unworthily</u> can be the cause of your sickness, so asking God's forgiveness for partaking previously unworthily will completely erase the unfortunate event from God's mind[1]. Now taking communion correctly from now on will ensure long life, health, and prosperity. As you see above in verse 28, you are to "examine yourself" prior to partaking of communion. The word "examine" is the Greek word, *dokimazo*, which by definition means, "to prove by test, put to the proof, examine; especially metals etc., by fire, and of other things by use; to examine, judge of, estimate; *hense* approve by trial[2]." So, as you can see, you must perform a self-test. This testing is defined in the content of the chapter as to whether you are in fellowship and are one with the Body of Christ. 'When you receive Jesus you are in Him and He is in you and the Body of Christ is the church with Christ as the head and the members fulfilling their unique function. You cannot be wishy-washy as to being a part of the Body. If you cut off your hand by accident, the hand will surely die if a surgeon cannot reconnect it to your body. The severed hand may continue to look like a hand for a while, but soon it will wither and disintegrate. You cannot be "outside" of the Body of Christ Jesus and live. You may still look like a member of the Body, you may still even go to church…but the consequences apparently are that your physical body will become weak, sick, and eventually die.

- **"Second Aid"** is your pastor, or minister. Many times someone with a deeper knowledge of spiritual matters is required. They can give crucial guidance and have insight into the knowledge of God's Word concerning your issues. Healing and true cures are available. Remember the examples in the Bible. When Jesus Christ and the disciples were able to perform great signs, miracles and healings, it was when they accessed God's holy power. The times the disciples could not heal the people is when they, or the people had no faith. You still have to believe for healing. Believing is an action word. It is just like the man with the crippled hand. Jesus said, "Stretch forth thy hand," When the man acted on the command and stretched forth his hand, his hand then was healed, not before that time. You can't go to your minister or pastor and put the responsibility on them for your healing. You must be actively involved. If you have to keep reminding yourself to believe –

you're not believing. When you are really believing, it is not an issue.

- **"Third Aid"** is where you have used first and second aid and still need to find help from a knowledgeable healthcare practitioner. This is the correct order of things. If you have a deep splinter in you, you could by faith have it disappear. However, a doctor can easily remove it thereby allowing it to heal. Many people are afraid of the alternative therapies due to lack of understanding, and their desire not to do anything contrary to God's Word. I do encourage you to find a Christian healthcare provider. Keep in mind that a hammer is a great tool if you want to build a house, but if you use it to hit someone in the head and kill them…is it less of a tool? Most healing remedies and techniques are tools which when used correctly can aid in facilitating correction by your body. It is always your body that does the healing. No one tool can correct all of the problems in the body. If you have a worm in your liver, I can not give you a chiropractic adjustment and correct that problem. However, if you dislocate your finger there is no pill that I could give you to put the finger back. The more tools your doctor has to facilitate the healing of your body the more likely your recovery. Homeopathy can be a wonderful tool to facilitate the correction of long forgotten issues. Professional Christian psychotherapists are another avenue available. Myofascial therapies can many times bring out in the open, stored emotional issues that can be like a poison to the body slowing the healing process. Keep in mind that when your body sees that someone is helping things, your body will naturally begin to bring things off the back burner to be finally dealt with. You may see many odd and unexplainable problems suddenly show up out of the blue. Your body really desires to be rid of all of the garbage.

Chapter 7

What to Expect with Alternative Medicine

If you are suffering from any chronic illness it is almost a given that you have had "suppressive" therapies used on you. For example: if you went to your doctor for headaches, what would the doctor usually give you? A painkiller most likely...after all, you are having a headache due to the fact that your body is deficient in aspirin, right? Wrong answer! The headaches continue to worsen until the aspirin no longer works, so your doctor puts you on something stronger. The cause of the headache remains untouched. You just can't feel it. All you are doing is buying yourself time. You will have to "pay the piper" eventually when all of the different painkillers don't even affect the headaches anymore. Always remember that true healing cannot occur by simply masking the symptoms.

Alternative medicine practitioners attempt to address the <u>cause</u> of the headaches. The relief is sometimes as quick or quicker than drug painkillers. Sometimes when you choose alternative medicine for chronic illnesses, you may feel worse before you feel better. This is good in most cases, because it means that the causes of your symptoms, instead of the symptoms only, are finally being addressed. Some people call this a "healing crisis", but a thoughtful planning of treatment by your physician can limit the severity of the problems. Over-aggressive treatment will undoubtedly cause more severe healing crises.

Feeling worse during treatment happens because so much of what is wrong in your body are things that your body has adapted to. If you do not get the appropriate treatment when something goes wrong, then your body is forced to adapt and get used to things being out of place and out of balance. When your doctor begins to correct these issues, the body will bring all of these problems "off the backburner" to be dealt with. Many times you will find that you retrace your steps chronologically. The most recent problem will be the first to go, while the first or initial problem to show up will be the last to go. Once you realize that this is what is happening you can rejoice, because you know where you are in your healing. If you stop treatment half way through this chronological retracing you can already know much of what you have to look forward to in the upcoming months and years, since you've already been there.

The following protocol was designed to limit and hopefully eliminate any "healing crisis" by effectively addressing the needs of the body in states of chronic illness.

Do not be afraid. It took a long time to get to this point, and it is going to take time to heal as well. As a general rule, you should allow three months of proper treatment for every year you have had your condition. Every single atom of your body is replaced at least one time per year. It takes about six weeks for the bottom layer of skin to become the top layer. Old skin cells are constantly dying and being replaced by new ones. You get a new liver however only once in four months. The goal is to remove the problems that are causing the perpetuation of dysfunctional cells so that when the body replaces cells it is able to replace them with good healthy cells. Nerve tissue takes the longest to regenerate. So, do not look at this illness as a possible quick fix situation. It is going to take good therapies that do not harm the body and a whole lot of time.

Keep in mind, that so many symptoms are blamed on Lyme Disease, when the fact of the matter is that it may be something entirely different causing some of your symptoms. Parasites, non-related bacterial and viral infections, systemic yeast infections, toxic overload, and poor lifestyle choices can be the cause of some of your symptoms. This is one of the strengths of our treatment protocol outlined here; it addresses many of these common problems.

Chapter 8

A Comprehensive Treatment Plan

<u>A comprehensive treatment plan should at least include the following:</u>

- Address each of the Borrelia burgdorferi life-stages...
- Address any other concomitant viral, mycoplasmal, fungal, and bacterial infections.
- Eliminate complicating factors...candidiasis (systemic yeast infection), parasites (intestinal, organ, or blood parasites), poor circulation, increased toxic load.
- Create avenues of elimination and detoxification.
- Re-establish total body ecology...acidophilus, pH balancing, dietary counseling based on blood type.
- Increase tissue nutritional support.
- Address any mental, emotional, geopathic, barometric, or miasmic stress.
- Remove nerve interference with chiropractic care and establish proper bio-mechanical and bio-electrical issues.
- Re-establish proper rhythm in your body with cranial-sacral technique.
- Re-establish your innate electrical energy with acupuncture.

Surviving chronic Lyme Disease is not inexpensive.
The very nature of the illness demands only the best of therapies. In light of the fact that as a nation we spend a disproportionate amount of money on health in the last three months of our life, it makes more sense to not just do the minimum to achieve optimum health today. The following is what I consider to be an optimum protocol. The remedies recommended are the best the world has to offer at this time, in my opinion.

THE OPTIMUM PROTOCOL

Essential Survival Support:

- **Borrelogen**...a complex botanical medicine, primarily anti-spirochetal in action. This herbal formula has been designed to be of specific benefit to those suffering from chronic Lyme Disease, Babesiosis, Ehrlichiosis, Chronic Fatigue Syndrome, Multiple Sclerosis, Lupus, ALS, Fibromyalgia, and/or Mastocytosis. Borrelogen is a unique proprietary formula containing extracts of Phragmites Communis Rhizome, Morus Alba leaf, Fiddle-leaf fig folium, Chrysanthemum moritolium flower, Platycodon grandiflorum root, Prunum armeniaca kernel, Glycerrhiza uralensis root, Baptisia australis, Mentha hapocalyx, Ophiopogon tuber, Una-de-gato, Morus rubra fruit, Cuscuta, Scindapsus aureus, Ipomoea quamoclit. It is essential to combine Borrelogen with Virogen for maximum synergistic effect when suffering from chronic Lyme Disease. This product has been tested by independent laboratory and found to be non-toxic at a dose of 150 times the maximum recommended adult dosage[1-2].

- **Virogen**... Virogen herbal formulation was developed using a technique called Bio-Resonance Scanning (BRS) to help maintain a healthy body in individuals suffering from chronic L Form, viral, and mycoplasmal type infections. Virogen contains extracts of three unique herbs, which have never before been used in this combination. The herbs, *Cuscuta sp.* and *Calvatia sp.* have been used for over 5000 years while the ipomea quamoclit is a relative newcomer. It is recommended especially for those suffering from Lyme Disease, Gulf War Illness, Multiple Sclerosis, Rheumatoid Arthritis, Lupus, Chronic Fatigue Syndrome, Fibromyalgia, Mastocytosis, Herpes virus, colds, flus and any suspected viral condition. It is essential to combine Borrelogen with Virogen for maximum synergistic effect when suffering with <u>chronic</u> Lyme Disease.

- **Monolaurin**...Monolaurin is an exciting product because its antiviral properties enable selective use of an agent which is non-toxic to humans. Monolaurin works directly on the envelope coat of the virus. By disrupting the conformation of this lipid bilayer, Monolaurin prevents attachment (absorption) to susceptible host cells. Clinical studies have shown that Monolaurin is effective against Herpes I & II, Epstein-Barr virus, Influenza and cytomegalovirus (CMV), all of which share lipid envelope characteristics. Included in this group is the HTLV virus, which is trophic towards T-cells. In studies performed at the Respiratory Virology Branch, Center for Disease Control, Atlanta, Georgia, Monolaurin was tested for virucidal activity against 14 human RNA and DNA-enveloped viruses in cell culture. Monolaurin removed >99.9% or all measurable infectivity of the 14 viruses by disintegrating the virus envelope. The viruses used were prototype or recognized representative   strains of enveloped human viruses obtained from the reference virus collection at the CDC [3-10].

- **Artemesia Annua**... pharmacological and clinical research has shown an inhibitory effect *in vitro* against many common dermatomycoses and leptospirosis. It has also shown a direct killing effect against the malaria parasite *in vitro*. It can be beneficial for low fevers, improved digestion, headache, rashes, dizziness, stifling sensation in the chest, nosebleeds, useful in liver and gallbladder, and is widely known to be antiparasitic[11-12].

- **Germanium Sesquioxide**…a trace element of profound importance which appears to be highly effective in stimulating electrical impulses on a cellular level. Also known as Organic Germanium, it increases the oxygen-carrying ability of the blood. Every atom of Germanium carries four oxygen atoms into the bloodstream. Germanium is believed to be the active ingredient in many popular herbs such as, Garlic, Aloe, and Ginseng. Reported to help relieve pain. Organic germanium is believed to help your body discharge unwanted electrical current, and to allow much needed current to flow through, thereby establishing the desired electrical balance. It restores the normal function of T-cells, B-lymphocytes, antibody-dependent cell toxicity, natural killer cell activity, and the numbers of antibody-forming cells… all this without any significant toxic effects[13].

- **Yeast Ease**…an herbal combination containing Maclura pomifera leaf extract and Illinois bundleflower seed extract. Yeast Ease assists the body in maintaining proper body ecology in regards to systemic candida populations. Independent laboratory in vitro testing of Yeast Ease has verified that even when diluted at 1:800 with water it still achieves a significant 80% reduction in Candida albicans, the most common form of chronic yeast infections. Also, following FDA guidelines, independent lab testing has determined that Yeast Ease is non-toxic[15]. Independent laboratory testing demonstrated significant effectiveness for the five most common strains of candida yeast[16]. This product has been tested by an independent laboratory and found to be non-toxic at a dose of 150 times the maximum recommended adult dosage.

- **Molybdenum Chelate**… A trace mineral which is an essential part of at least 3 key enzyme systems and supports the liver's detoxification of sulfites (in many preservatives), alcohol (in beverages and medications), aldehydes (a toxic byproduct of candida yeast die-off and other various chemicals), and copper containing compounds[17]. Many reports verify its benefit in relieving much of the yeast and bacterial "die-off" symptoms called Jarish-Herxhiemer Reactions.

- **Paragen**…an herbal tincture of Maclura pomifera fruit extract to promote the elimination of intestinal and blood parasites. It aids in re-establishing proper pH levels in the intestines. It improves absorption of nutrients and also beneficial in normalizing bowel movements. Parasites can cause body aches and pains remote to their location. It is effective for: constipation, diarrhea, colic, stomach cramps, anemia, malnutrition, joint pain, acidosis, toxemia, nausea, vertigo, dizziness, eye problems, ear aches, attention deficit disorder, miscarriages, birth defects, leaky gut syndrome, irritable bowel disease, liver dysfunction, excessive mucus, respiratory problems, unexplained fevers, and the list could go on and on.

- **Joint-Aide**…Nutritional support for the soft-tissues and cartilage of the body. Helps reduce joint pain, swelling and restricted motion. It is also beneficial in irritable bowel, and leaky gut syndrome. Joint-Aide includes glucosamine hydrochloride, Boswella, Sea Cucumber and essential vitamins and minerals for maximum utilization by the body.

- **CoQ_{10}**…essential for generating energy. Plays an important role in your body's antioxidant system. This product is mixed with Vitamin E and rice bran, which in combination can significantly reduce free-radical damage in the liver, kidney and heart tissues. Another beneficial role of CoQ10 is to increase macrophage activity.

- **Bio-Thymic Protein A**…Research has verified that this is one of the best products to stimulate the immune system. The thymus is your body's immune-system regulator. The thymus gland is the activator of T-lymphocytes, cells that play an essential role in the body's defenses against infections. This thymus extract stimulates your thymus to produce 60 different hormone-like polypeptides which act as messengers, instructing T-cells to fight infection. Normally the older one gets; the smaller and less active the thymus becomes.

- **High Delivery Acidophilus**...Eight different strains of beneficial intestinal friendly acidophilus bacteria. Helps in the replacement of friendly flora after antibiotic. Research has demonstrated that acidophilus type bacteria help to control the over-population of candida type yeast.

- **SeaSilver**...Liquid food-form nutrition...provides at the cellular level every vitamin, macro mineral, trace mineral, amino acid, and enzyme known to man in food form balance. This is not a mega-vitamin, it provides the nutrients your body needs using proprietary processing methods to increase the bio-availability for maximum digestion, absorption, and assimilation of all nutrients at the cellular level. I like SeaSilver because as a liquid your body does not have to break down a tablet in order to receive benefit. Also, many of my patients have chronic malabsorption syndrome as a result of their long fight with infection and they can not digest tablets efficiently. From my clinical experience this product is "slurped up" by the body and the benefits are happening as soon as it hits your mouth.

For obvious reasons, the following does <u>not</u> claim to substitute for a physician's care, nor does it advocate specific solutions to individual problems. These products and the information below should not be regarded as a substitute for professional medical treatment.

General Recommendations for the Use of Supplements

I would recommend staying on this protocol until your symptoms have been relieved and stay gone for at least four months. Use half the indicated amounts for children under the age of 10, or as directed by your physician.

- Borrelogen..........32 drops, 3 times per day under the tongue, or in water or juice.
- Virogen............ 32 drops, 3 times per day under the tongue, or in water or juice.
- Artemesia Annua extract..32 drops, 3 times per day in water or juice.
- Monolaurin..........1 – 300 mg capsule, 3 times per day.
- Yeast Ease.........32-64 drops, 2-3 times per day under the tongue, or in water or juice.
- Paragen.............32 drops, 2-3 times per day under the tongue, or in water or juice.
- Joint-Aide..........2-3 capsules, 2-3 times per day.
- Germanium.........1 - 150 mg capsule, 3 times per day.
- CoQ10..............1- 100 mg gelcap, 2-3 times per day with meals.
- Bio-Thymic Protein A...1 packet under tongue for 5 minutes, 1 time per day.
- Molybdenum.......1 – 300 mcg tablet, 3 times per day. (Do not exceed this amount)
- Acidophilus.........1 capsule, 2 times per day (2,000 mg/day)
- SeaSilver............1 fl.oz., 2 times per day undiluted or in purified water.
- Purified water......64 fl.oz. per day

Chapter 9

Beneficial Survival Support

- **Detox/Pain-Relieving Baths**...these baths are believed to be beneficial in assisting your body in eliminating toxins. Studies have shown that some people have been able to get off of their pain medicines with this bath therapy. See *Appendix*.
- **Glyconutritionals**...These molecules are required for cell-to-cell communication and identification. The only company I recommend is the Mannatech Company, which produces an outstanding patented product, called Ambrotose.
- **Deep Breathing**...The lungs are a part of the body's detoxification system. As you exhale, you are ridding your body of toxins, as you inhale deeply you are increasing your body's available oxygen. Try doing a minimum of 10 minutes of quiet deep breathing.
- **Eat According to your Blood-type**...Definite must read, *"Eat Right for Your Type"* by Dr. Peter J. D'Adamo. This astounding research based book has shaken the world! Prior to this research, the dominant opinion was that everyone should only eat fresh fruits and vegetables. Now it has been eloquently demonstrated that a more accurate way to eat is based on your Blood-type (O, A, B, AB) For example...Wheat is basically a poison for

persons with Blood-type O, who do better with eating specific types of meat.

- **Different Bodies, Different Diets**…A detailed guidebook with 25 body types so that you can determine more accurately the type exercise needed, types of food required, and on which meals to focus to build your immune system. One volume for men and another for women, a textbook for building a healthy body individualized to each person. Written by Dr. Carolyn Mein, D.C.

- **Balance Total Body Ecology**…Another book that is a must read! *"Body Ecology"* by Donna Gates. Only by eliminating all harmful factors in your life and balancing your body's ecology from every angle will your reality of life be improved. Do not completely rely on pills, drugs, or supplements to heal you.

- **Eliminate All Toxic Products from your House**…Most household cleaners, soaps, detergents, air-fresheners, disinfectants, toothpaste, cosmetics, bug sprays, and the like, are known to contain toxins which are bio-accumulative. These toxins are absorbed by the body in minute amounts, but accumulate in the body's tissues to harmful levels over time. We are in a sea of petroleum based products which are very harmful. You must source reduce. Get rid of the source of the toxins in your life. Replace your toxic products with brands known for their safety and non-toxic ingredients. I recommend the Melaleuca brand cleaning products. I have seen the MSD sheets (Material Safety Data sheets) – required by the government to list all ingredients' safety, on these products and believe them to be better than most. Most of the products have no toxic ingredients and are very beneficial to overall health due to the healing properties of the Tea Tree Oil in the products. The Weleda Company, established in 1921 in Switzerland, provides what I consider to be the finest, most effective, all natural, toxin-free personal care products.

- **Get a Biological Dentist to Check Your Dental Work**..."Dental factors have been associated not only with the cause but also with the cure of chronic disease." Also research has demonstrated that "factors contributing to chronic degenerative diseases include energy blockages and toxicity from mercury amalgam dental fillings. Symptoms ascribed to mercury toxicity include fatigue, depression, anorexia, insomnia, arthritis, moodiness, irritability, memory loss, nausea, diarrhea, gum disease, swollen glands, and headaches, among others." Published studies have reported reversal of illness in such cases as Multiple Sclerosis, Alzheimer's, Cancer, Arthritis, and Parkinson's. Read: *The Key to Ultimate Health*, by Ellen Hodgson-Brown and Richard T. Hansen, DDS.

Chapter 10

What Kind of Doctor Should I Go To?

I highly recommend that you seek out a doctor who is willing to treat you as a totally integrated organism. The human body is reliant on each tissue functioning properly in order for long term health to be achieved. All it takes is one organ to malfunction to cause a chain reaction of other glands and organs to become effected over time.

Ideally you should see an M.D. that can provide you with the prescription medicines you may need and one who will work in tandem with an allied health professional who is proficient in Applied Kinesiology, Electro-dermal testing, or Clinical Kinesiology. These treatment techniques are now accepted worldwide. They are very beneficial in that they all help to eliminate some of the guesswork of doctoring. The best of all worlds would be an M.D. who uses the above techniques and recognizes that the ideal is to treat the patient naturally and completely, not just with pills and IVs. Doctors using these techniques or other variations can test your body's responses to whatever therapy you choose to determine if you actually need the remedy, will be allergic to it, or have become toxic to it. What you pay most doctors for is their best educated guess. The products I am recommending here are a collection of the best remedies I know of for spirochete sufferers based on the Bio-Resonance Scanning technique I have used for many Lyme sufferers.

I <u>want</u> you to have these remedies tested by a doctor practicing one of the above techniques! Don't take my word for it! These doctors can tell you whether the remedies will helpor not, based on their testing methods. Most, if not all of the doctors who have tested our products using these methods agree that they are very beneficial and effective. None of the remedies listed have been reported to aggravate conventional antibiotic therapies.

The primary philosophy of this alternative medicine protocol is to assist your body in eliminating the bottom-line problems and to provide your body with the building blocks it needs to heal itself. Mark my words, if you have to keep taking a product forever to feel good, or any time you have to take a medicine forever to keep your body working correctly, then it is not addressing the bottom-line problem, it is just masking the symptoms. True healing cannot occur by simply masking the symptoms! The ultimate goal is for your body to finally function correctly the way it was designed to without having to take anything other than proper nutrition.

Chapter 11

The Electrical Organization of Your Body

You are one organism. You are not a collection of unrelated pieces and parts. Every tissue of the body is energetically linked together in complex electrical circuitry[1]. You might think of the circuits in your house as an analogy. Your house doesn't have just one circuit, if it did you would be constantly blowing the fuse from the overload and demand on the circuit. A circuit in your house is an electrical path of dedicated wiring that may have a light switch, three different light fixtures and the wiring on it. The body also has many different electrical circuits. A circuit in your body includes a specific set of teeth, one organ, at least one muscle type, and the electrical "wiring" or nerve pathways that supply the circuit with electricity.

The circuits in the body can also be likened to a string of Christmas lights...if one bulb blows the whole string goes. If there is any problem in a circuit of the body, the entire circuit will "blow" and the available electricity in the circuit will be reduced to about 40% of what it should be. This happens so that you cannot hurt yourself by using 100% of your energy on a "broken" part. With only 40% of the energy you can still function and you can do so without hurting yourself seriously. This is a protective mechanism of your body. If you literally tore a muscle in half due to an accident, your body would protect you from tearing it the rest of the way by turning down the available electricity to that muscle so that you couldn't use the muscle as strongly.

Most people have not had the benefit of being treated in such a way as to keep all of the body's circuits up and running. Because of this we usually see that by the age of 20, the vast majority of people have twenty or more body circuits functioning at only 40%. This is due to the fact that if one circuit becomes dysfunctional or has an unresolved problem, it causes a chain-reaction of other circuits that become affected over time. As the body compensates for the problem, the organs and tissues on the different circuits exceed their design specifications and one by one become dysfunctional.

To say that someone has 20-25 different circuits blown means that there are at least 25 different sets of muscles that are only working at about 40% of their ability. Folks, you can work these muscles out at the gym all year and they may get stronger, but they will still only be getting proportionately 40% of the juice to them. Can you see why chronic weakness and fatigue is such a problem in Lyme Disease?

In the house scenario, if you go to turn on the lights and they don't come on, at that point you don't know what the problem is. The symptom is that the lights will not come on. If the cause of the problem is in the light switch, then you can put in new light bulbs, you can replace the light fixtures, you can put gold plated wiring in, but it will never get the lights to come on again. You must address the bottom line problem, the light switch. It is the same in the body! Your doctor must identify all of the bottom line problems, not just the bacteria, and he must get all of the circuits of the body up and running again.

Isolating and testing the strength of each individual muscle can quickly assess the integrity of the different circuits. When a doctor challenges the resistance strength of a muscle, the muscle should catch and hold rigid with 100% electricity getting to it. If the muscle is spongy when challenged, it would demonstrate that there is something wrong in the circuit and only 40% of the electricity is in the circuit.

If the muscle tests weak and spongy feeling, at this point we still do not know what has gone wrong in the circuit. It could be a problem in the muscle, the organ may be damaged from infection or toxins, the tooth may be compromised from infection or mercury from silver amalgams[2], or possibly the electrical and nerve pathways are damaged from degeneration. A well-trained doctor has ways to further test to determine where the problem is in the circuit. Once the bottom line problem is identified a correction can be made and the circuit will come back to 100% and the muscle will test strong and firm.

Keep in mind that the electricity of your body is not "all or none" electricity like the electricity of your lights, where they are either on or off. The electricity of your body we now know has the ability to carry an infinite amount of information. It is your brain's way of communicating to over 50 trillion cells how to function and repair themselves. Without the full 100% of the electricity flowing through each circuit the brain cannot effectively and completely heal your body.

Most people will live out their entire life on "secondary wiring", the 40% electrical capacity. Since the beginning of time, doctors have never been able to test so accurately as the present advanced Bio-Resonance and kinesiology testing. You can live to be over 100 years of age on secondary wiring, but at the sacrifice of quality of life. I encourage you to find a doctor knowledgeable in this type of treatment. It could be that your infection is gone, but the "lights are not on" that is keeping you from realizing great health.

Chapter 12

Beneficial Therapies

Oxygen Therapies

One of the characteristics unique to the L Form of Lyme borreliosis and mycoplasma is their absolute anaerobic nature. Optimum growth occurs in an environment of no oxygen. (CWD) This vulnerability to oxygen can be used to suppress these infections[1].

There are a number of ways to increase oxygenation of the body:

1. Pulsed Magnetic Field Therapy
2. Hyperbaric Oxygen Chamber
3. Microcurrent Therapy
4. Hydrogen Peroxide Bath Therapy
5. Various Nutritional and Mineral Supplements.
6. Moderate Aerobic Exercise
7. Breathing Exercises

Ideally you should combine all of the above therapies in the proper sequence to achieve maximum oxygenation of the tissues.

Pulsed Magnetic Field Therapy (PMFT)

PMFT is new to the United States with only eight units being used by doctors in the States at the time of this writing. This machine was developed in Germany and has a very impressive track record, benefiting illness ranging from sinusitis to arthritis, diabetes, circulatory problems and even cancer. Doctors and patients report high success rates among the more than two million patients already treated in hospitals, pain clinics, and practices in Europe. More than 60,000 treatments with PMFT are done on a daily basis. There are no known side effects or contraindications with PMFT.

Pulsating magnetic fields penetrate the body completely. Every cell in the body is exposed, even into the bone and bone marrow.

A direct result of applying PMFT to tissue, is a change in oxygen partial-pressure (pO2), and this is of importance for all tissues, but is of major importance for body parts supplied with oxygen through diffusion, such as cartilage and the vertebral discs of the spine.

The change in the partial-pressure of oxygen means that there is an increased movement of oxygen through the tissues and an increased utilization of oxygen in the cells, which increases the energy metabolism.

The entire body can be influenced bioenergetically by the physical dimension "magnetic field" at a certain frequency and intensity. It is known that in different diseases the electrical resting and threshold potentials of cells differ from normal values, thus impairing the cell function. With PMFT, the ions present in the cells and in the colloidal system are magnetically influenced. As they are exposed to the pulsating magnetic fieldlines of a specific frequency, the ions are pressed against the cell membrane producing a hyperpolarization, which has a positive influence on the intracellular metabolism, particularly on the energy metabolism. If this procedure is applied over a determined period of time, it leads to a normalization of the electrical potential difference. As a result there is improved ion dynamics at the cells' interface, resulting in the increased utilization of oxygen in the cell. This increases the production of energy for healing and overall cellular function, in the form of ATP (adenosine triphosphate). The resultant increase in ATP from using PMFT can be measured.

PMFT and ATP and Chronic Illness

ATP, adenosine triphosphate, is one of your body's primary energy molecules that is produced by every cell for every day functioning and for healing. ATP is produced by the mitochondria, the energy factories in every cell. You burn up to 40% of your total body weight in ATP every day. This means that if you weigh 100 pounds, you are using up 40 pounds of ATP every day. Thankfully you can recycle the resultant ADP (Adenosine Diphosphate) that way you don't just disappear completely in about three days! Below you will see how this 40 pounds of ATP is used in your body. Its use can be broken down into thirds, so consider as in the above 100 pound person, 13.3 pounds of ATP is being used every day for the following three general ways.

ATP use can be broken down into three major functions:

- ATP production is extremely important especially in Lyme Disease, because one-third of all of the ATP produced in your body is used to pump out the sodium from the neurons via the sodium/potassium pumps. In states of chronic illness the body's metabolism becomes compromised and the energy production in the form of ATP, slows down. Without enough ATP to pump out the sodium from the nerve fibers, the nerve fibers begin to degenerate. As degeneration of the nerve occurs you experience tingling, muscle weakness, numbness, and the ultimate progressive dysfunction of multiple organ systems. So, you can see the importance of your doctor maintaining or re-establishing the ATP production of your body.
- One third of the ATP your body produces is used to facilitate enzyme reactions. If the body's enzyme reactions do not have the ATP to function correctly, many of the chemical reactions in the body will not happen quickly enough to be of any good. This enzymatic breakdown leads to multi-system dysfunction affecting all aspects of sense of well being and strength. PMFT increases

the metabolism (all of the chemical reactions occurring in the body) by hyperpolarizing the cells which is beneficial in turning up the ATP production for these enzymatic/chemical reactions.

- The last third, or 13.3 pounds, of the ATP is used for energy to run all of the contractile muscles and non-contractile tissues of the body. In this area ATP shortage is noticed most remarkably in muscle fatigue and atrophy. When all is functioning correctly, the muscle fibers are "pumped up" from weight bearing exercise and the muscle fibers are filled with energy producing mitochondria which are little organs inside of the cells that are simply ATP factories. When multiple systems become dysfunctional and multiple electrical circuits are "blown" the demand for energy is great, but the body is unable to generate the electricity it needs to keep the mitochondria working. One by one the mitochondrial energy factories shut down, ATP production falls sharply and the muscle atrophies or shrinks in size and strength. In order for PMFT research to demonstrate an increase in ATP, it must be re-energizing the mitochondrial energy factories.

Your body's metabolism becomes sluggish during chronic illnesses and ATP production goes down because the demand for energy wanes as the cells become *hypo*functional. The mitochondrial energy factories gradually begin to shut down to just a "skeleton crew" and only enough mitochondrial energy factories remain to barely "keep the lights on". To say that a therapy increases the production of ATP means that the energy factories are fired up again in response to reinforcement from the cells becoming less hypofunctional and more functional again.

A healthy functioning cell needs a lot of energy and can get it when all the players are present and working. Once there is enough ATP the body can get busy repairing, replacing, and rebuilding. As the tissues become healthier, the body's natural resistance to infection is re-established and with other appropriate treatments such as antibiotics the infections can be completely eliminated.

PMFT is only now getting a foot-hold in the United States, but research has been ongoing in Europe and around the world using this particular device for the last 25 years.

Apart from many other diseases, Pulsating Magnetic Field Therapy may be applied with great therapeutic success in the following ailments:

- Diseases of the support and locomotor system, particularly rheumatic and arthritic disorders.
- Sports injuries such as bruises, pulled or torn ligaments and muscles, tennis elbow.
- Delayed wound healing and non-union fractures.
- Headaches and migraines
- Heart and circulatory diseases, circulatory disturbances
- Metabolic disorders
- Neuralgia
- Bronchitis and sinusitis, acute and chronic

It stands to reason that many of the above ailments known to respond well to PMFT, are now becoming known to be caused by infectious anaerobic organisms. One can see the truth in the ability of the PMFT to increase the oxygenation of the tissues thereby assisting in the killing of anaerobic microbes.

When used in conjunction with Hyperbaric Oxygen Therapy (HBOT) a synergistic effect is achieved enabling deeper penetration and utilization of the oxygen into all the cells of the body. PMFT is a strong stand-alone therapy, but it will also enable you to get more out of your HBOT treatments.

The really nice thing about this therapy is that it is relatively inexpensive, especially when compared to Hyperbaric Oxygen treatments.

Hyperbaric Oxygen Therapy

Hyperbaric oxygen (HBOT) is a therapy which allows patients to breathe 100% oxygen through a hood or mask while in a compressed air chamber. Such exposure results in a large increase in the partial pressure of oxygen in the plasma and subsequently delivers increased oxygen to the tissues.

HBOT BENEFITS
1. Hyperoxygenation of the blood
2. Fibroblast Proliferation and Enhanced Function
3. Neovascularization
4. Antimicrobial action of high oxygen
5. Enhancement of leukocyte functions
6. Vasoconstriction
7. Enhancement of some antibiotic activity
8. Compression of bubbles

There are many benefits to using HBOT, but the primary benefits to someone suffering from Lyme Disease are listed below:
1. Hyperoxygenation of the blood elevates the amount of dissolved oxygen and results in the correction of tissue hypoxia (Decreased available oxygen in the tissues of the body). This results in improved or enhanced wound healing, and infection control.
2. Direct toxicity to anaerobic bacteria (bacteria that cannot live in an oxygen rich environment). The second method of infection control is through an indirect effect by the enhancement of white blood cell killing of phagocytized bacteria. Elevated oxygen increases the oxygen free radicals and hydrogen peroxide formation in the white cell lysosomes, improving their antimicrobial activity.
3. In inflamed and swollen, or edematous tissue, HBOT leads to constriction of hypotonic blood vessels which can reverse the fluid loss into the tissues and reinstate normal lymphatic drainage. Also, HBOT appears to improve capillary integrity reducing the leakage that causes edema.
4. Selected medicines become more effective with normalization of tissue oxygen or high partial pressure of oxygen.

One of the most important roles of oxygen in wound healing is its contribution to the immune response to infection. It is well known that leukocytes require oxygen in order to kill efficiently. In a hypoxic wound, a wound that has little or no oxygen getting to it, HBOT increases oxygen tension in tissue, thus providing the essential substrate for the oxygen dependent leukocyte intracellular killing mechanisms.

Chapter 13

"No Brainer" Things To Do

1. Ladies, if you are using the birth control pill, you need to seriously think about finding an alternative contraceptive because of the intense strain birth control pills place on your body. Consider Natural Progesterone cream if you are having PMS, menstrual irregularities, menopausal symptoms, or energy and sleep problems. Proper hormone balance can make all the difference in your healing. Read... *What Your Doctor May Not Tell You About Menopause*, by John R. Lee, M.D. Even if you are a woman in your early twenties you may benefit more than you could imagine from this book. Dr. Lee has recently written another book entitled *What Your Doctor May Not Tell You About Premenopause*. We recommend the Natural Woman® Natural Progesterone cream, because it has the highest amount of natural progesterone per jar at 960mg. Beware of some herbal wild yam creams, which according to Dr. Lee have little or no actual natural progesterone.

2. Avoid MSG (monosodium glutamate)...This is a flavor enhancer type food-additive. Read labels on foods and spice packs. This substance is known as a central nervous system Excitotoxin. Glutamate crosses the blood-brain barrier irritating brain function and peripheral nerve tissues. Read *Excitotoxins*, by Russell L. Blaylock.

3. Avoid NutraSweet®…another excitotoxin to the brain and nervous system. A bi-product of NutraSweet® is wood alcohol, which is widely known to be very toxic to the human body. (NutraSweet® company is now in court fighting lawsuits due to the epidemic of problems being blamed on this substance) Read *Excitotoxins*, by Russell L. Blaylock.

4. Increase your water intake…purified water is a must, because of the documented impurities, parasites, and viruses known to permeate municipal water. Although drinking three quarts of water per day will not flush out the Lyme bacteria, it will flush out many of the toxic byproducts that cause pain in the body. Keep in mind that water is required for every single chemical reaction in the body. Drinking coffee, teas, or juices can not substitute for water, because it requires all of the water in the coffee, tea, or juice to process those substances out of the body. Drinking these will actually create a water deficit, or dehydration since many of these drinks have diuretic (stimulates urination) actions.

5. Absolutely no soda, pop, colas or whatever you want to call them. Most of these drinks have as much as six tablespoons of sugar in a 12 oz. can. The sugar literally burns up the islets of Langerhan in the pancreas, the cells responsible for producing insulin. Eventually enough of these cells are lost and hypoglycemia turns into diabetes. Many of you have chronic fatigue as a component of the LD. Get off of the sugar roller coaster. Stevia is an herbal sweetener that can be found in many health food stores that is a much safer sugar substitute than the other artificial sweeteners. It is totally safe for diabetic people.

6. Eliminate all milk and dairy products. This may be too drastic for many of you, but you should be told anyway. "A sip of milk contains hundreds of different substances, each one having the potential to exert a powerful biological effect when taken

independently of the others. Pus, blood, feces, allergenic proteins, naturally occurring powerful growth hormones, fat, cholesterol, pesticides with vitamin D added, viruses, bacteria (including bovine leukemia, bovine tuberculosis and bovine immunodeficiecy virus) all combine to produce a vast array of ailment in our society", according to researcher Robert Cohen. Lyme Disease is a war...dairy products act as glue in your body's war machine. Dr. Julian Whitaker, MD is the founder and editor of the largest read health newsletter in the world. Dr. Whitaker agrees that you should "knock off drinking milk altogether", and to "use all dairy products sparingly, and be sure to avoid products from hormone-treated cows." If you want to learn more concerning this matter read the book, *Milk, The Deadly Poison*, by Robert Cohen.

7. If you are doing something obviously bad...STOP! These are things like smoking, chewing tobacco, drinking alcohol, taking recreational drugs, eating junk and chemically dead foods, and the like.

Chapter 14

40 Thoughts To Live By

1. In times of change, learners will inherit the earth, while the learned will find themselves beautifully prepared to deal with a world which no longer exists.

2. What you say, and what you think, is every cell's command – be sure the commands you are sending are not perpetuating the illness.

3. It's not "all in your head", but illness requires your head to be into and inline with your healing.

4. Determine and focus your mind on your body as you would have it be, and then never waver from that image. Your body will hear the command and make it so.

5. Focus on the illness and it will grow; focus on healing and it will be.

6. Doctors can help your body to heal, but only you can give your body the permission to heal totally.

7. What you need to learn is to never speak a negative. When you have a problem, never tell more people than necessary – your brain is listening.

8. This is a law of nature: Believing = Receiving, whether negative or positive.

9. Believe that you will be completely well again the way you believe that the letter you just mailed will actually reach its destination, or the way that you believe that the Statue of Liberty is in New York even though you may have personally never seen it.

10. In dealing with pressure, you have to realize that all pressure begins in the mind. You allow yourself to be pressured.

11. To speed healing, you must get the hurt and dirt out of your life.

12. Change involves work.

13. You will never get the answer to a question you never ask.

14. Truth is truth, come hell or high water.

15. Truth is forever on the scaffold.

16. Where knowledge fails, heart sustains.

17. Negatives are like mosquitoes on a blood hunt.

18. All strain is drain.

19. Positive thoughts combat negative thinking.

20. Thinking patterns determine your heart, your heart determines your health.

21. Be patient with yourself.

22. Don't sacrifice your whole life because you have a wound in one area.

23. You do your best. Trust God to do the rest.

24. Action cures fear. Non-action strengthens fear.

25. Be an active participant in your own healing.

26. What you are doing today will determine your tomorrow.

27. It's really not how long we live that counts, but the quality of our lives while we are living.

28. The more work you have to do, the more disciplined you have to be to get the desired work done.

29. You are the sum total of the decisions you've made.

30. Abundance is not a state of being, but a state of mind.

31. The greatest part of education is learning to think for yourself.

32. I see my life far beyond today and tomorrow. I see my life from generation to generation causing them to live a stronger heritage.

33. We plant the trees so that someone else may enjoy the privilege of sitting in the shade.

34. I wish I were the man I know to be; however, I always strive to do better.

35. Minds are like parachutes: they work best when they are open.

36. Why continue to go to the world for answers when it's the world that confused you in the first place?

37. One must be as willing to unlearn as to learn.

38. All life is dependent upon decision; accomplishment is attained by carrying out that decision.

39. Be assured of this...you never have a headache due to a deficiency of aspirin.

40. Looking back gives you a stiff neck.

Chapter 15

Research On Borrelogen

Acute Oral Toxicity Test – ISO

ISO is designed to assess the acute oral toxicity of test substance, Borrelogen, occurring within 14 days of the oral administration of a single dose or multiple doses of the test substance administered within 24 hours.

The test substance, Borrelogen, was evaluated for its potential to produce death following oral administration at a dose of 2 grams/kilogram of body weight in male and female Sprague-Dawley rats. Based on the absence of mortality and the criteria of the study protocol, *the test substance is defined as nontoxic.* This study was conducted in compliance with the U.S. Food and Drug Administration (FDA) regulations set forth in 21 CFR, Part 58 and OECD GLPs, current version. The sections of the regulations not performed by or under the direction of Toxikon Corp, exempt from this Good Laboratory Practice statement, include characterization and stability of the test and its mixture with carriers, 21 CFR, Part 58.105, and 58.113. The assessment of an LD_{50} was not necessary. No toxicity was observed in post study necropsy of the different organ systems[1].

Borrelia burgdorferi Antigen Release Stimulation by Nutraceutical Formula as Determined by Lyme Urine Antigen Testing

It is understood that antigens are the cause of numerous sensitivities resulting in much of the symptomatology experienced in chronic illness. This clinical study was restricted to determining whether Borrelia burgdorferi specific antigen could be purged from circulation by the use of a nutraceutical formula called Borrelogen. The results are very preliminary as more research is needed to rule out physiological interference. LUAT assay was utilized to determine antigen release after 68 subjects used the nutraceutical for one week. Results revealed 73% of the subjects released specific antigen to the degree of being considered positive or highly positive by LUAT. (Only seventeen of the 68 subjects were tested by Lyme Western Blot IgM/IgG prior to starting Borrelogen. All seventeen subjects were either Equivocal or Positive via this serological assay.) This study in itself cannot be used to make definitive statements about the efficacy of Borrelogen, only that an antigen was released from whatever mechanism. Note: IGeneX is not in any way endorsing this nutraceutical, nor is IGeneX associated in anyway with Jernigan Nutraceuticals Inc. IGeneX was blinded to the use of the nutraceutical and only performed the testing procedure. True research seeks to find the truth in an unbiased manner for the betterment of mankind.

Introduction

Bacteria contain many particulate and soluble antigens that evoke strong, often lasting immune responses, both humoral and cellular.[2] According to Stedman's Medical Dictionary, an antigen (allergen); is any substance that, as a result of coming into contact with appropriate tissues induces a state of sensitivity.[3] Antigens are understood to cause many of the symptoms experienced by LD sufferers. It would stand to reason that decreasing the antigen load on the body would correspondingly decrease the number and severity of symptoms.

A proprietary nutraceutical formulation was developed in 1998 to specifically target the functional release of spirochetal antigen from the tissues of the body. The historical and pharmacognostic data of the individual plant-based extracts reveal very low toxicity, while being functionally beneficial in many ways to the body.

The research presented here was performed as a clinical study to aid in our understanding of the potential effectiveness of the nutraceutical formula, Borrelogen™. Lyme Urine Antigen Testing (LUAT) was chosen as a viable determinant due to its specificity to Borrelia burgdorferi antigens seen as a result of a release of antigen from an appropriately applied therapy. Because the body will as a natural process release Lyme specific antigen in about **30%** of untreated cases, the nutraceutical formula was tested to see if the body could be stimulated to release a greater amount of antigen, with a higher percentage of positive LUATs.

A nutraceutical is defined as a plant-based remedy that is specifically formulated to target specific body dysfunctions.[4]

Methods

Participants in this study were pre-selected based on positive Borrelia burgdorferi screening using a neurological sensory-based, Bio-Resonance Scanning™ assay. The group consisted of 68 people residing in a non-endemic area of the United States. All were suffering from a range of 3 to 44 chronic problems based on a 55 question Lyme Disease symptom questionnaire.

Lyme Urine Antigen Testing (LUAT) was utilized to monitor the release of antigen. LUAT testing is an antigen capture assay specific to detection of low levels of antigen, in spite of the presence of other proteins. The antibody being used in this antigen capture is a unique polyclonal antibody that is specific for the 31 kDa (OpsA), 34 kDa (OpsB), 39 kDa, and 93 kDa antigens of Borrelia burgdorferi. This assay appears to be very specific to these antigens with a reported false positive rate of less than 1% in a study of 408 controls.[5]

The reference range of a LUAT is based on P-values or confidence levels. Antigen levels reported as ≥32 ng/ml have a 95% confidence level of being positive and distinguishable from a negative population.[3]

A LUAT is a highly controlled and reproducible assay which is used in conjunction with patient history, symptoms and serum panels. The nice thing about LUAT assay is that it is positive throughout all three stages of infection: early, which is said to be <60 days (which is before you normally can get a seropositive result); second stage, which is defined as 60 – 360 days; and the third stage >360 days.[6]

Results

Reporting only the highest score of the three-day urine collection the majority of positive LUATs scored over 100 ng/ml. Out of the 68 LUATs performed 44 were reported as positive or highly positive, while there were 4 borderline, and 18 negative results. The total percentage of positive scores was 73%. When the nutraceutical formula was used instead of prescription antibiotics the majority of positive LUATs were reported over 100 ng/ml, and as high as >400 ng/ml. Although a score of >400 does not indicate that a patient is more highly infected than a score of >45, it does indicate a high rate of antigen release which can only benefit the patient. An interesting side-note, only seventeen of these 68 cases were also tested by Lyme Western Blot IgM/IgG prior to taking the Borrelogen. All seventeen subjects tested as positive or equivocal by Lyme Western Blot.

Conclusion

Based on this study, it appears that this nutraceutical formula does indeed stimulate the purging of Borrelia burgdorferi antigens from the body. This antigen-detox can only be seen as a good thing as these antigens when circulating throughout the body cause a multitude of systemic sensitivities, which in turn causes increased suffering in the patient. An infected person does not release antigens daily or uniformly.[7] The fact that in this study, 73% of the time when using this nutraceutical a high release of antigen was stimulated is significant.

Further research must be performed to determine if a negative control group on the same protocol would yield a similar effect. However, based on positive patient symptomatic response and clinical observations we are encouraged that this botanical formula may effectively stimulate and increase the tissue elimination of deleterious antigen via the urine. Further research may also result in increased probability of highly positive Lyme Urine Antigen Test confirmations.

Interference studies performed by IGeneX lab confirmed that Borrelogen does not cause a false positive LUAT when negative patient urines were spiked in various concentrations. This *in vitro* assay does not, however, effectively rule out the possibility of *in vivo* interference.

Chapter 16

Miasms - What makes you tick?

Did you ever wonder why you act the way you do, or why you suffer with certain types of illnesses? How you act and the things you suffer from may have more to do with your ancestors than with your lifestyle. The theory of Miasms may explain some of what makes you tick. This is not "new age" and is not genetic abberations, but is more of an energetic phenomenon.

A miasm, by definition, is a predisposition, or tendency to certain psychological and physical problems that you either inherited or acquired within your own lifetime[1-2]. Miasms are not to be confused with genetic abnormalities, such as missing or mutated genes. Miasms are more of an energetic abnormality. John Davidson, a researcher and author on bioenergetics, states that "miasms are essentially an energy disharmony, dis-ease pattern or imbalance."

Research dating back over 200 years document the reality of these energetic problems. Miasms are usually started by improperly treated illnesses that can go back as far as seven generations of your family tree. In other words, some of the tendencies you have, could be the result of illnesses your parents had, or medications they took before you were born, or even by your great, great...grandparents' illnesses[2].

For over two hundred years, scientists have been tracking the miasms caused by specific illnesses. Today we have immense collections of data outlining what kinds of problems future generations may experience due to different illnesses. Gonorrhea, syphilis, tuberculosis, cancer, and many more, all will generate a specific set of problems unique to the illness when suppressive therapies are used to treat them. Antibiotics are a suppressive therapy and, some agree, are the major culprit to creating miasms. The antibiotics do kill the bacteria that cause these different illnesses, but they do nothing to address the damage already done by the bacteria on a physical and bio-electrical level in the patient's body. For example, if you find that you have termites in you house, you can call an exterminator to come out and kill the termites. By killing the termites you have made it where the problem should not get worse, however, you have done nothing to correct the myriad of tunnels through the woodwork of your house. To make matters worse, you now have a very toxic chemical insecticide in your house. These tunnels and toxins, in a nutshell, are what cause miasms to occur.

How are miasms passed from generation to generation?
When a girl or boy is born, they carry the family blueprints in their eggs and sperm. These blueprints are being constantly modified. You might say it is an ongoing project that is passed on to each new generation. My sperm carry the blueprints unique to the Jernigan family. When combined with my wife's blueprints each generation puts in their two cents worth on how the child should be made. Throughout both sets of blueprints there are energetic flaws, miasms, which out of the ignorance of past doctors went uncorrected. The union of these blueprints results in a child. This child came to this world created with his or her unique set of blueprints. Let us assume for the sake of demonstration that this is a boy child whose parents got properly treated and passed on no miasms. His blueprints have no flaws. The years go by and he gets an ear infection, which due to social pressures, the parents have treated with antibiotics. Instantly, the blueprints in the little boy's sperm are modified. His sperm will now create offspring that may have tendencies to similar problems i.e. ear infections and the psychological problems unique to the miasm. The boy will live through these minor illnesses.

The boy grows up and for example's sake we'll say he is sexually promiscuous, before he is married, and catches gonorrhea. This is a major miasm. Gonorrhea, and the standard treatment, cause major modifications to his blueprint in the sperm. He later settles down and marries a nice girl. This is where it really gets interesting – keep in mind that the blueprint in the sperm is being modified bio-electrically (or energetically).

Can a Miasm be sexually transmitted?

When the above couple has sexual intercourse the man's sperm is deposited within the woman. Research has verified that the sperm are viable up to three days, so for three days the woman is forced to integrate some of the miasmic energy of the sperm! In a bizarre way the woman becomes linked to that man energetically. This may be some primeval mechanism to ensure the procreation of the species, much like the way many birds and animals mate for life. It may also ensure that miasmic corruption of blueprints is kept to a minimum – possibly such as inbreeding problems seen in the breeding of purebred dogs. It is theorized that this may also be why some wives continue to stay with a husband who physically and emotionally abuses them.

Even if this couple never has children, the woman will suffer primarily on a psychological level because of the miasmic transfer from the husband's sperm. It is primarily on the psychological level since it is the most vulnerable to energetic change, however over the course of many years the woman may experience physical symptoms as well, caused purely by the miasm.

If this couple were to have children, the father's miasm-damaged blueprint would be passed on to the child, predisposing the child to similar problems and tendencies which, if left untreated, will be passed on for another 5 generations.

What if a woman has had multiple sex partners?

In theory, each man's sperm can adversely affect the woman on a miasmic level. This may be one reason why most religions adhere to the belief that one should wait until marriage to have sexual intercourse.

Like father, like son!

The Bible even mentions that the sins of the father are passed on through the blood seven generations. So, the next time you hear someone say, "I'm just like my Mom, a worrier", or "I have my Dad's hot temper", or "Everyone in my family has diabetes", you can recognize it for what it really is – a miasm.

Marriage Concerns

I know it is not romantic, but you should be concerned about your potential spouse's family health history. If nothing else you and your significant other should be treated before you start a family.

How are miasms corrected?

The only recognized way to effectively eliminate existing miasms is with the proper homeopathic remedy. Normally only one to three doses is necessary to remove the miasm from the blueprint. "Energy is never lost, only transformed or relocated and homeopathic cure attempts, therefore, to smooth out the disharmony of the miasm, as the basic cause of disease…The release of the entire miasmatic trait would result in a complete cure… If therefore, a miasm is successfully treated, the energy field is re-polarized."[2]

The best way to avoid acquiring new miasms is to combine the proper homeopathic remedies with whatever other treatments you choose. Only a doctor trained in homeopathy, or a professional homeopath trained in the treatment of miasms should address these types of issues.

Chapter 17

Don't Get Ticked

Proper Tick Removal

(Reprinted with Permission from the Lyme Disease Foundation)

1. Use a fine-point tweezer to grasp the tick at the place of attachment, as close to the skin as possible.
2. Gently pull the tick straight out.
3. Place the tick in a small vial labeled with the victim's name, address, date, and estimated hours attached.
4. Wash your hands, disinfect the tweezer and the bite site.
5. Call your doctor to determine if treatment is warranted.
6. Have the tick identified/tested by a lab, health department, or veterinarian.

To Protect Your Family

(Reprinted with permission from the Lyme Disease Foundation)

- **Wear light-colored clothes** when you venture into grass, woods, garden or beach areas so you can more easily see the ticks. Tuck shirt into pants and pants into socks to thwart a tick's effort to crawl under your clothing and get to your skin.
- **Avoid tick-infested areas**, avoid sitting directly on the ground, and stay in the center of paths.
- **Use EPA-approved tick repellants.** Once inside, wash off repellants.
- **Do frequent tick-checks**, including a naked, full body exam upon returning inside.

Chapter 18

Tracking Your Symptoms

Use this helpful listing of symptoms to monitor your progress. Using a scale of 1 - 10, with 10 being your absolute worst, and 1 being no problem; write the number that most accurately describes your condition, try to be as objective as possible since this can help you see your improvement.

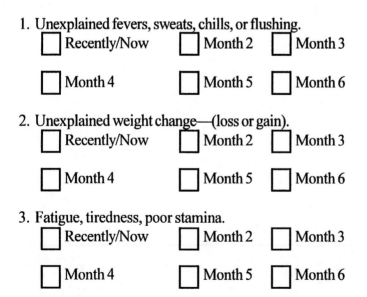

1. Unexplained fevers, sweats, chills, or flushing.
   ☐ Recently/Now   ☐ Month 2   ☐ Month 3

   ☐ Month 4   ☐ Month 5   ☐ Month 6

2. Unexplained weight change—(loss or gain).
   ☐ Recently/Now   ☐ Month 2   ☐ Month 3

   ☐ Month 4   ☐ Month 5   ☐ Month 6

3. Fatigue, tiredness, poor stamina.
   ☐ Recently/Now   ☐ Month 2   ☐ Month 3

   ☐ Month 4   ☐ Month 5   ☐ Month 6

4. Exhaustion upon awakening
☐ Recently/Now ☐ Month 2 ☐ Month 3

☐ Month 4 ☐ Month 5 ☐ Month 6

5. Very nervous—laughs or weeps without cause
☐ Recently/Now ☐ Month 2 ☐ Month 3

☐ Month 4 ☐ Month 5 ☐ Month 6

6. Unexplained hair loss
☐ Recently/Now ☐ Month 2 ☐ Month 3

☐ Month 4 ☐ Month 5 ☐ Month 6

7. Swollen glands
☐ Recently/Now ☐ Month 2 ☐ Month 3

☐ Month 4 ☐ Month 5 ☐ Month 6

8. Sore throat
☐ Recently/Now ☐ Month 2 ☐ Month 3

☐ Month 4 ☐ Month 5 ☐ Month 6

9. Testicular pain/pelvic pain
☐ Recently/Now ☐ Month 2 ☐ Month 3

☐ Month 4 ☐ Month 5 ☐ Month 6

10. Upset stomach
☐ Recently/Now ☐ Month 2 ☐ Month 3

☐ Month 4 ☐ Month 5 ☐ Month 6

11. Change in bowel function—(constipation, diarrhea)
☐ Recently/Now   ☐ Month 2   ☐ Month 3

☐ Month 4   ☐ Month 5   ☐ Month 6

12. Chest pain or rib soreness
☐ Recently/Now   ☐ Month 2   ☐ Month 3

☐ Month 4   ☐ Month 5   ☐ Month 6

13. Shortness of breath, cough
☐ Recently/Now   ☐ Month 2   ☐ Month 3

☐ Month 4   ☐ Month 5   ☐ Month 6

14. Heart palpitations, pulse skips, heart block
☐ Recently/Now   ☐ Month 2   ☐ Month 3

☐ Month 4   ☐ Month 5   ☐ Month 6

15. Any history of a heart murmur or valve prolapse?
☐ Recently/Now   ☐ Month 2   ☐ Month 3

☐ Month 4   ☐ Month 5   ☐ Month 6

16. Joint pain or swelling
☐ Recently/Now   ☐ Month 2   ☐ Month 3

☐ Month 4   ☐ Month 5   ☐ Month 6

17. Muscle pain or cramps
☐ Recently/Now   ☐ Month 2   ☐ Month 3

☐ Month 4   ☐ Month 5   ☐ Month 6

18. Unexplained menstrual irregularity
- [ ] Recently/Now
- [ ] Month 2
- [ ] Month 3
- [ ] Month 4
- [ ] Month 5
- [ ] Month 6

19. Disorientation: getting lost, going to wrong places.
- [ ] Recently/Now
- [ ] Month 2
- [ ] Month 3
- [ ] Month 4
- [ ] Month 5
- [ ] Month 6

20. Dyslexia
- [ ] Recently/Now
- [ ] Month 2
- [ ] Month 3
- [ ] Month 4
- [ ] Month 5
- [ ] Month 6

21. Difficulty processing auditory or visual information
- [ ] Recently/Now
- [ ] Month 2
- [ ] Month 3
- [ ] Month 4
- [ ] Month 5
- [ ] Month 6

22. Difficulty with speech or writing
- [ ] Recently/Now
- [ ] Month 2
- [ ] Month 3
- [ ] Month 4
- [ ] Month 5
- [ ] Month 6

23. Mood swings, irritability, depression
- [ ] Recently/Now
- [ ] Month 2
- [ ] Month 3
- [ ] Month 4
- [ ] Month 5
- [ ] Month 6

24. Symptoms worse from alcohol
- [ ] Recently/Now
- [ ] Month 2
- [ ] Month 3
- [ ] Month 4
- [ ] Month 5
- [ ] Month 6

25. Disturbed sleep—too much, too little, early awakening
- [ ] Recently/Now
- [ ] Month 2
- [ ] Month 3
- [ ] Month 4
- [ ] Month 5
- [ ] Month 6

26. Ears/Hearing: buzzing, ringing, ear pain, sound sensitivity
- [ ] Recently/Now
- [ ] Month 2
- [ ] Month 3
- [ ] Month 4
- [ ] Month 5
- [ ] Month 6

27. Increased motion sickness
- [ ] Recently/Now
- [ ] Month 2
- [ ] Month 3
- [ ] Month 4
- [ ] Month 5
- [ ] Month 6

28. Lightheadedness, wooziness
- [ ] Recently/Now
- [ ] Month 2
- [ ] Month 3
- [ ] Month 4
- [ ] Month 5
- [ ] Month 6

29. Tremors
- [ ] Recently/Now
- [ ] Month 2
- [ ] Month 3
- [ ] Month 4
- [ ] Month 5
- [ ] Month 6

30. Confusion, difficulty thinking
- [ ] Recently/Now
- [ ] Month 2
- [ ] Month 3
- [ ] Month 4
- [ ] Month 5
- [ ] Month 6

31. Difficulty with concentration, reading
- [ ] Recently/Now
- [ ] Month 2
- [ ] Month 3
- [ ] Month 4
- [ ] Month 5
- [ ] Month 6

32. Stiffness of the joints, neck, or back
- [ ] Recently/Now
- [ ] Month 2
- [ ] Month 3
- [ ] Month 4
- [ ] Month 5
- [ ] Month 6

33. Twitching of the face or other muscles
- [ ] Recently/Now
- [ ] Month 2
- [ ] Month 3
- [ ] Month 4
- [ ] Month 5
- [ ] Month 6

34. Symptoms worse at night
- [ ] Recently/Now
- [ ] Month 2
- [ ] Month 3
- [ ] Month 4
- [ ] Month 5
- [ ] Month 6

35. Bone pains
- [ ] Recently/Now
- [ ] Month 2
- [ ] Month 3
- [ ] Month 4
- [ ] Month 5
- [ ] Month 6

36. Despair of recovery
- [ ] Recently/Now
- [ ] Month 2
- [ ] Month 3
- [ ] Month 4
- [ ] Month 5
- [ ] Month 6

37. Tail bone pain on sitting
- [ ] Recently/Now
- [ ] Month 2
- [ ] Month 3
- [ ] Month 4
- [ ] Month 5
- [ ] Month 6

38. Difficulty raising arm laterally or in front
- [ ] Recently/Now
- [ ] Month 2
- [ ] Month 3
- [ ] Month 4
- [ ] Month 5
- [ ] Month 6

39. Sciatica
- [ ] Recently/Now
- [ ] Month 2
- [ ] Month 3
- [ ] Month 4
- [ ] Month 5
- [ ] Month 6

40. Unexplained milk production
- [ ] Recently/Now
- [ ] Month 2
- [ ] Month 3
- [ ] Month 4
- [ ] Month 5
- [ ] Month 6

41. Breast pain
- [ ] Recently/Now
- [ ] Month 2
- [ ] Month 3
- [ ] Month 4
- [ ] Month 5
- [ ] Month 6

42. Sexual dysfunction or loss of libido
- [ ] Recently/Now
- [ ] Month 2
- [ ] Month 3
- [ ] Month 4
- [ ] Month 5
- [ ] Month 6

43. Irritable bladder or bladder dysfunction
- [ ] Recently/Now
- [ ] Month 2
- [ ] Month 3
- [ ] Month 4
- [ ] Month 5
- [ ] Month 6

44. Headaches
- [ ] Recently/Now
- [ ] Month 2
- [ ] Month 3
- [ ] Month 4
- [ ] Month 5
- [ ] Month 6

45. Vertigo, dizziness, poor balance
- [ ] Recently/Now
- [ ] Month 2
- [ ] Month 3
- [ ] Month 4
- [ ] Month 5
- [ ] Month 6

46. Eyes/Vision: double, blurry, increased floaters, light sensitivity
   ☐ Recently/Now   ☐ Month 2   ☐ Month 3

   ☐ Month 4   ☐ Month 5   ☐ Month 6

47. Difficulty processing auditory or visual information
   ☐ Recently/Now   ☐ Month 2   ☐ Month 3

   ☐ Month 4   ☐ Month 5   ☐ Month 6

48. Facial paralysis (Bell's Palsy)
   ☐ Recently/Now   ☐ Month 2   ☐ Month 3

   ☐ Month 4   ☐ Month 5   ☐ Month 6

49. Soreness of the chest
   ☐ Recently/Now   ☐ Month 2   ☐ Month 3

   ☐ Month 4   ☐ Month 5   ☐ Month 6

50. Chronic asthma worse at night
   ☐ Recently/Now   ☐ Month 2   ☐ Month 3

   ☐ Month 4   ☐ Month 5   ☐ Month 6

51. Dry cough worse at night
   ☐ Recently/Now   ☐ Month 2   ☐ Month 3

   ☐ Month 4   ☐ Month 5   ☐ Month 6

52. Neck creaks and cracks, neck stiffness, neck pain
   ☐ Recently/Now   ☐ Month 2   ☐ Month 3

   ☐ Month 4   ☐ Month 5   ☐ Month 6

53. Tingling, numbness, burning, or stabbing sensations
- [ ] Recently/Now
- [ ] Month2
- [ ] Month3
- [ ] Month 4
- [ ] Month 5
- [ ] Month 6

54. Great restlessness at night- absolute sleeplessness after Midnight
- [ ] Recently/Now
- [ ] Month 1
- [ ] Month3
- [ ] Month4
- [ ] Month 5
- [ ] Month6

55. Diagnosis of an auto-immune disease - Multiple Schlerosis, ALS, Lupus, Fibromyalgia
- [ ] Recently/Now
- [ ] Month 2
- [ ] Month 3
- [ ] Month 4
- [ ] Month 5
- [ ] Month 6

56. Forgetfulness, poor short-term memory
- [ ] Recently/Now
- [ ] Month 2
- [ ] Month 3
- [ ] Month 4
- [ ] Month 5
- [ ] Month 6

57. Chest pain or rib soreness
- [ ] Recently/Now
- [ ] Month 2
- [ ] Month 3
- [ ] Month 4
- [ ] Month 5
- [ ] Month 6

References

Chapter 2

1. Mattman, L., Cell Wall Deficient Forms, Stealth Pathogens, 2nd Ed. 1992

2. Per telephone conversation with Dr. Lida Mattman Ph.D, July, 1999.

3. Mattman, L., Cell Wall Deficient Forms, Stealth Pathogens, 2nd Ed. 1992

4. Cotran, Kumar, Robbins. *Robbins Pathological Basis of Disease.* 4th Edition

5. Mattman, L., Cell Wall Deficient Forms, Stealth Pathogens, 2nd Ed. 1992

6. Murphy R, Lotus Materia Medica, Lotus Star Academy Publishing, 1995.

Chapter 3

1. Mattman, L., *Cell Wall Deficient Forms, Stealth Pathogens,* 2nd Ed., p 13, 1992

2. Popular Science, April 1999

3. Donta, S. T., *Fibromyalgia, Lyme Disease, and Gulf War Syndrome*, 12th International Conference on Lyme Disease, New York, 1999

4. Nicolson, G.L., Nasralla, M, Hier, J. and Nicolson, N.L. Mycoplasmal infections in chronic illnesses: Fibromyalgia and Chronic Fatigue Syndromes, Gulf War Illness, HIV-AIDS and Rheumatoid Arthritis. Med. Sentinel 1999.

5. Nicolson, G.L, The Institute For Molecular Medicine, 1999.

Chapter 4

1. A Novel Toxin (Bb Tox 1) of Borrelia burgdorferi, Mark J. Cartwright, Ph.D.

2. Martin, S.E, Donta, S.T., International Conference on Lyme Disease, New York, April, 1999.

3. The Physician's Clinical Reference Manual, Cass, R., 1994, p. 112

Chapter 5

1. Coyle, P. K., Neurologic Lyme Disease Update, International Conference on Lyme Disease, New York, 1999.

Chapter 6

1. Psalms 103:12, Micah 7:19, Hebrews 8:12, Hebrews 10:17.

2. Bullinger E W, *A Critical Lexicon and Concordance to the English and Greek New Testament*, Zondervan Publishing, 1975.

Chapter 8

1. Benesky/Gamble, *Materia Medica, Chinese Herbal Medicine*, Eastland Press 1993.

2. Duke JA, Foster S, Eastern/Central Medicinal Plants, Houghton Mifflin Press 1990.

3. Cohen, S.S. *Strategy for the chemotherapy of infectious diseases*. Science 197;431, 1977.

4. Dulbecco, R. *Interference with viral multiplication*. Virology, Harper & Row, Philadelphia, 1980.

5. Kabara, J. J. *Fatty acids and derivatives as antimicrobial agents*. Antimicrob. Agents Chemother. 2;23, 1972.

6. Kabara, J. J. *Lipids as host-resistance factors of human milk*. Nutr. Rev. 38;65, 1980.

7. Hierholzer, J. C. et al. *In vitro effects of Monolaurin on enveloped RNA and DNA viruses.* J. Food Safety, 4:1, 1982.

8. Sands, J. A. et al. *Antiviral effects of fatty acids and derivatives.* Pharmacological Effects of Lipids. Am. Oil Chem. Soc.: Champaign, 1979:75.

9. Sands, J. et al. *Extreme sensitivity of enveloped viruses, including herpes simplex, to long-chain unsaturated monoglycerides and alcohols,* Antimicrobial Agents and Chemotherapy, 15(1):67-73, 1979.

10. Kohn, A. et al. *Unsaturated free fatty acids inactivate animal envelope viruses*. Arch. Virol. 66:301-306, 1980.

11. Leung A, Foster S. Encyclopedia of Common Natural Ingredients Used in Food,   Drugs, and Cosmetics, 2nd Ed. New York: John Wiley & Sons, 1996, 1-3.

12. Benesky/Gamble, *Materia Medica, Chinese Herbal Medicine*, p. 110, Eastland Press 1993.

13. Kamen, B., *Germanium, A New Approach to Immunity*, Nutritional Encounter Publishing, 1987.

14. Walter LD, Elvin-Lewis M, *Medical Botany*, John Wiley & Sons, 1977.

15. Shwaery, G.TPh.D., 99G-0905, 1999 Toxikon Corp. / International Nutraceutical Research Group, 1999.

16. Great Smokies Reference Laboratory, North Carolina / International Nutraceutical Research Group, 1999.

17. Cass, R., The Physician's Clinical Reference Manual, p. 112, 1994.

Chapter 11

1. Becker, R. O., The Body Electric, Electromagnetism and the Foundation of Life, Quill Publishing, 1985.

2. Brown, J. D., Hansen R T, The Key to Ultimate Health, Advanced Health Research Publishing, 1998.

Chapter 12

1. Intern. J. Medicine 1998; 1:123-128.

Chapter 15

1. Glenn T. Shwaery, G.TPh.D., 99G-0905, 1999 Toxikon Corp. Sponsored by International Nutraceutical Research Group.

2. Cotran, Kumar, Robbins. Robbins Pathological Basis of Disease. 4th Edition; p.335.

3. Stedman's Medical Dictionary. 25th Ed. Williams & Wilkins

4. Journal of Nutraceuticals and Functional Foods, 1994.

5. Callister SM, Schell RF. Laboratory Serodiagnosis of Lyme Borreliosis. J Spirochetal Tick-borne Inf 1998;1: 21.

6. Harris NS. IGeneX Reference Laboratory Guide. 1998; 4.

7. Harris NS, Stephens BG. Detection of Borrelia burgdorferi Antigen in Urine from Patients with Lyme Borreliosis. Journal of Spirochetal Tick-borne Inf. 1995; 2: 41.

Chapter 16

1. Murphy, R., Lotus Materia Medica, Lotus Star Academy Publishing, 1995.

2. Davidson, J., Subtle Energy, p. 222-28, C W Daniel Co, 1993.

Appendix A

Recommended Reading

-*Different Bodies, Different Diets, Dr. Carolyn Mein, D.C.*

-*Eat Right for Your Type,* Dr. Peter J. D'Adamo, N.M.D.

-*Excitotoxins, The taste that kills*, Russell L. Blaylock, M.D.

-*The Body Ecology, Recovering Your Health & Rebuilding Your Immunity*, Donna Gates

-*Germanium, A New Approach to Immunity*, Betty Kamen, Ph.D.

-*What Your Doctor may not Tell You About Menopause*, John R. Lee, M.D.

-*Cell-Wall Deficient Bacteria, Stealth Pathogen,* Lida Mattman, Ph.D.

Appendix B

Protocol Product Information

Ancient Formulas
638 W. 33rd St. N.
Wichita, Kansas
800-543-3026

Products: Joint Aide

Ecological Formulas
1061-B Shary Circle
Concord, California 94518
800-888-4585

Products: Monolaurin

Energique Inc.
P.O. Box 121
Woodbine, Iowa 51579
800-869-8078

Products: High Delivery
Acidophilus,
Artemesia

Healing Within
84 Berkeley Ave.
San Anselmo, California 94960
800-300-7548
www.healingwithin.com

Products: CoQ^{10}, Virogen,
Bio-Thymic High Protein
A, Borrelogen, Paragen,
Artamesia

Jernigan Nutraceuticals
3621 E. Kellogg Drive
Wichita, Kansas 67218
888-456-8872
www.jnutra.com

Products: Borrelogen,
Monolaurin, Virogen,
Organic Germanium,
Molybdenum, Paragen

SeaSilver Inc.
P.O. Box 189002
Carlsbad, California 92009
1-800-299-8256

Products: SeaSilver

Appendix C

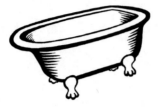

Detox/Pain-Relieving Bath Recipe

2 cups of Epsom Salts
3 32oz. Hydrogen Peroxide 3%
1 tsp. grated fresh Ginger (Optional)

Add all ingredients to hot bath water (not too hot) and soak your body for at least 20 minutes. (Research shows that you reach the maximum benefit from bath therapy at 20 minutes of soaking.)

Many people stop here, but it would enhance your body's response to inflammation to follow with a cold shower. This bath should be free from soaps and other body products. This bath can be taken 1-2 times daily, or as needed. It may take a few baths for the full benefit to kick in.

Appendix D

Internet Resources

Lyme Disease Foundation
   www.lyme.org

Lyme Disease Network
   www.lymenet.org

American Lyme Disease Foundation
   www.aldf.com

Center for Disease Control - Lyme Disease Site
   www.cdc.gov/ncidod/diseases/lyme

Lyme Alliance
   www.lymealliance.org

Lyme Disease in the United States & useful links
www.geocities.com/HotSprings/Spa/6772/lyme.html

National Center for Homeopathy
   www.healthy.net/nch

Eat Right For Your Type - Dr. D'Adamo
   www.dadamo.com

Alternative Medicne Practitioners Directory
   www.altmedweb.com

IGENEX Reference Laboratory
   www.igenex.com

HealthWorld Online - Free Medline
   www.healthy.net

Appendix E

Lyme Literate Doctors
Using Alternative Medicine

The following doctors are included in the listing by their request and permission. The treatment methods used address the complete body, not just an illness or infection.

Alabama
> Holistic Healing Arts Center
> Karen Kelley, N.M.D., D.C.
> 10200 County Rd. 65 S.
> Foley, AL 36534
> 334-943-8883

California
> Spectrum Health Center
> Randy March, D.C.
> 900 Fulton Ave., Ste. 300
> Sacramento, CA 95825
> 916-482-4150

Connecticut
> Kathleen M. Riley, N.M.D.
> 31 Hawleyville Rd.
> Hawleyville, CT 064403
> 203-426-2306

Georgia
> Rhett Bergeron, M.D.
> 320 Corporate Center Court
> Stockbridge, GA 30281
> 770-474-4422

Missouri
> Les Wilkie, D.C.
> 17701 E. 39th St., Ste. 100
> Independence, MO 64055
> 816-350-0999

Illinois
> Busse Wellness Center, Ltd.
> Susan Busse, M.D.
> Governors Place
> 2260 W. Higgins Rd.
> Hoffman Estates, IL 60195
> 847-781-7500

Kansas
> The Next Generation Wellness Center
> David A. Jernigan, D.C., B.S.
> 545 N. Woodlawn, Courtyard Ste.
> Wichita, KS 67208-3600
> 316-686-5900

New Mexico
> Gina Ogorzaly, D.C.
> 633 Kinley Ave.
> Albuquerque, NM 87102
> 505-242-1067

New York

Rhinebeck Health Center
Stephen Bock, M.D., Kenneth Bock, M.D.
108 Montgomery St.
Rhinebeck, NY 12572

Pennsylvania

First Health & Medical Center
Anthony Ferro, D.C.
1396 Wilmington Pike
West Chester, PA 19382
610-399-1900

Woodlands Healing Research Center
William Craght, D.O.
Henry Buttram, M.D.
5724 Clymer Rd.
Quakertown, PA 18951
215-536-1700

Wisconsin

Steven Bircher, D.C.
3321-A Golf Rd.
Eau Claire, WI 54701
715-832-1953

Glossary

Applied Kinesiology- A treatment technique used primarily by Doctors of Chiropractic, but also by some Medical Doctors, which uses a patient's neuro-muscular system to identify problem areas in the body to determine the most effective treatment. This type of treatment is very individualized to the patient and helps to eliminate guesswork on the part of the doctor.

Bio-Resonance Scanning- a neurological frequency matching system which allows the doctor to identify specific pathologies and determine appropriate treatments. This type of treatment is very individualized to the patient, and helps to eliminate guesswork on the part of the doctor.

Clinical Kinesiology- the offspring of Applied Kinesiology which is even more precise in determining not only what the patient's brain thinks is most important, but also uses the patient's brain as a bio-computer to determine the most effective treatments.

Electro-dermal Testing- this encompasses many different types of machines, which are usually computerized. Through meridian contact points, doctors can determine which systems of the body are being most stressed, what specific problems the body has, and which remedies will correct the problems.

Excitotoxins- a substance added to foods and beverages that literally stimulates neurons to death, causing brain damage of varying degrees. Can be found in such ingredients as monosodium glutamate (MSG), aspartame (NutraSweet®), cysteine, hydrolyzed protein, and aspartic acid.

Homeopathy- a form of medicine in which the "electrical signature" of a substance is harnessed and imprinted upon a carrier substance such as distilled water, or milk sugar crystals. Most homeopathic remedies contain no molecules of the original substance, but only carry the homeopathically modified electrical signature of that substance. "*Homeo,*" meaning similar and "*pathy*" meaning symptoms. By definition, a homeopathic remedy is a remedy which will create "symptoms" when repeated doses are given to a healthy individual. Conversely, for an unhealthy individual it will cure the symptoms.

Mycoplasma- a class of organism which is normally non-pathogenic. Its size is said to be in between that of a virus and a bacteria. Interestingly, the Gulf War Syndrome is causing many of the same symptoms as Lyme Disease and is now said to be caused by Mycoplasma fermentans incognitus.

Nutraceuticals- complex plant based medicines.

Pleomorphic- the ability of an organism to change shapes at different stages of its life. "*pleo*"- meaning "many"...and "*morph*" meaning "shapes". A butterfly is said to be pleomorphic in that it is a caterpillar, then a cocoon, then a butterfly.

Spirochete- a class of pathogenic bacteria typified by its spiral or corkscrew shape. Lyme Disease is caused by a spirochete called Borrelia burgdorferi.

Synergism- when two or more remedies complement the action of each other achieving a greater effect than using either one by itself.

About the Author

David A. Jernigan, D.C., B.S.

David A. Jernigan, founder of The Next Generation Wellness Centers and Chairman/CEO of Jernigan Nutraceuticals, is the developer of over thirty proprietary botanical and homeopathic medicines. As developer of Bio-Resonance Scanning, he lectures to doctors on this unique approach to identifying and treating various body malfunctions.

Other the years, Dr. Jernigan has seen the power of God manifested in knowledge and healing. He is greatly blessed by three children, and a loving wife, Dr. Sara Jernigan, D.C., B.S.

He is a graduate of Park College, Parkville, Kansas with a Bachelor of Science in Nutrition (with honors), and Cleveland Chiropractic College in Kansas City, Missouri where he received his Doctor of Chiropractic. Postgraduate studies include work with Hahnemann Academy of North America in homeopathy, University of Colorado School of Pharmacy in Botanical Medicine, and is currently Fellowship eligible with Open International Complementary Medicine University. In his leisure time, he enjoys hunting, sailing, and playing the Irish whistle.

Notes